FATTY LIVER COOKBOOK

MEGA BUNDLE – 3 MANUSCRIPTS IN 1 – 180+ Recipes designed to treat fatty liver disease

TABLE OF CONTENTS

BREAKFAST 12

SKINNY OMELETTE 12

VEGGIE QUINOA CUPS 13

CRANBERRY STUFFING 14

CRUSTLESS QUICHE CUPS 16

QUINOA WITH SCALLIONS 17

CORNBREAD MUFFINS 18

BERRY GRANOLA 20

OVERNIGHT OATS 21

TROPICAL OVERNIGHT OATS 22

DETOX GREEN MORNING SMOOTHIE 23

BERRY DETOX PORRIDGE 24

MORNING COOKIES 25

AVOCADO AND EGG TOAST 26

BREAFAST GLUTEN-FREE MUESLI 27

SWEET POTATO BREAKFAST WITH AVOCADO 28

MORNING BLACKBERRY COCONUT BOWL 29

COCONUT YOGURT WITH BERRIES 30

RASPBERRY SORBET 31

AVOCADO BROWNIE 32

BANANA PANCAKES 34

LUNCH 35

MINESTRONE SOUP 35

TUNA SALAD 36

CHICKEN SKILLET 38

SPINACH QUESADILLAS	39
BEAN SALAD	40
GARLIC SALMON	41
TUNA WRAP	42
ROASTED CHICKEN WRAP	43
LENTIL SALAD	45
STUFFED EGGPLANT	46
BROCCOLI & AURGULA SOUP	47
STUFFED PEPPERS	49
POTATO SALAD	50
PORK TACOS	52
CHICKEN & AVOCADO SALAD	54
PHILLY CHEESE STEAK	55
MAPLE-ROASTED SWEET POTATOES	57
MUSHROOM SOUP	58
DETOX SALAD	59
ROASTED ASPARAGUS	61
DINNER	62
GARLICKY TOFU	62
PORK MEATBALLS	63
ITALIAN PATE WITH FRIED ANCHOVIES	65
VEGETABLE FRITTATA	66
CHICKEN LIVER PATE	67
LAMB LIBERS WITH KALE AND LEMON	69
DANISH LIVER PATE	70
CHICKEN SALSA	71

SPAGHETTI SQUASH HASH BROWNS	73
BAKED PAPRIKA CHICKEN	74
CAULIFLOWER AND QUINOA SALAD	75
RASPBERRY BREAD	76
GREEK LAMB MEATBALLS	77
BAKED CHILLI CHICKEN	78
BROCCOLI STIR FRY	79
EGGPLANT FRIES	80
GLUTEN FREE BANANA CAKE	82
SEAFOOD CURRY	83
MASHED SWEET POTATOES	84
GARLIC SPICY CHICKEN	85
DESSERTS & SMOOTHIES	87
BLUEBERRY BITES	87
WATERMELON SMOOTHIE	88
GINGER LEMONADE	89
LIME GRILLED CORN	90
MOCKTAIL	92
BANANA MUFFINS	93
APPLE CRUMBLE	94
GINGERSNAPS	95
RICE KRISPIES	97
APPLE OATMEAL COOKIES	98
MINT CREAM	99
BLACK BEAN BROWNIES	100
TURMERIC TEA	102

PUMPKIN SPICE LATTE 103

GRANOLA 104

CHOCOLATE MOUSSE.. 106

ICED COFFEE 107

KALE ICE POPS 108

MACAROON BARS 109

CHOCOLATE ICE CREAM 110

FATTY LIVER DIET 112

50+ Side Dishes, Salad and Pasta recipes designed for Fatty Liver Diet 112

SALAD RECIPES 113

CHICKEN LIVER SALAD 113

SPICED CHICKEN LIVER SALAD... 114

CHICKEN LIVER AND BACON SALAD 115

CHICKEN LIVER SALAD WITH DRESSING 116

BUTTER & CAULI-COUSCOUS SALAD 117

LENTIL AND BRUSSELS SPROUT SALAD 118

CHICKEN CAESAR SALAD 120

CITRUS SESAME SEED SALAD 121

PROSCIUTTO SALAD WITH ORANGE VINAIRETTE........................ 122

COLESLAW 123

BLUE CHEESE AND FIG SALAD 124

VEGAN WHITE BEAN SALAD 126

JAPANESE VEGA SALAD DRESSING 127

ROASTED CAULIFLOWER SALAD.. 128

BROCCOLI SALAD WITH BACON 129

RED POTATO SALAD 130

TANGY RED CABBAGE SLAW 131
PIZZA RECIPES 133
GRAIN-FREE PIZZA CRUST 133
PIZZA WITH SPICY CHICKEN LIVER 134
DETOX CAULIFLOWER PIZZA 136
CAULIFLOWER CRUST PIZAA 137
LIVER DETOXIYING PIZZA 139
CAULIFLOWER PIZZA CRUST 141
EGGPLANT HUMMUS PIZZA 142
RAW SQUASH HUMMUS PIZZA 144
ZUCCHINI PIZZA CRUST 145
SPINACH PESTO PIZZA 147
RAW VEGAN PIZZA 148
SIDE DISHES 150
SESAME PORK TACOS 150
WATERMELON GAZPACHO 151
VEGETARIAN MINESTRONE SOUP 152
LIME GRILLED CORN 154
MACADAMIA DIP WITH VEGETABLES 155
GINGERSNAPS 156
TURKEY & VEGGIES STUFFED PEPPERS 158
QUINOA TACO MEAT 159
KALE CHIPS 161
CHICKEN AND BROWN RICE PASTA 162
PHILLY CHEESE STEAK 163
CAULIFLOWER WINGS 164

ROASTED BOK CHOY	166
ROASTED TURKEY	167
MAPLE-ROASTED SWEET POTATOES	168
CAULIFLOWER FRITTERS	169
PEACH CRUMBLE	170
GREEK MIXED VEGETABLES	171
CHICKEN BURGER	173
TURKEY MEATLOAF	174
PASTA & NOODLES	176
ROASTED CHICKPEAS	176
CHICKEN LETTUCE WRAPS	177
TURMERIC RICE	178
ROASTED BEET NOODLES WITH PESTO	179
AVOCADO PESTO NOODLES	181
BUTTERNUT SQUASH PASTA	182
LEMON PASTA WITH SHRIMP	183
FATTY LIVER DIET	185
50+ Smoothies, Dessert and Breakfast recipes designed for Fatty Liver Diet	185
BREAKFAST	186
PUMPKIN BAKED OATMEAL	186
BUCKWHEAT GRANOLA	187
FRUIT SMOOTHIE BOWL	189
BANANA PANCAKES	190
AQUAFABA GRANOLA	191
MORNING OATS	192
BANANA MUFFINS	194

CINNAMON PEANUT BUTTER 195

BANANA SPLITS 196

5 MINUTE RAW-NOLA 197

ZUCCHINI BREAD 199

PEANUT BUTTER & ACAI BOWLS 200

DARK CHOCOLATE GRANOLA 202

POTATO HASH BROWNS 203

BANANA NUT BUTTER PANCAKES 204

BREAKFAST MUFFINS 205

ZUCCHINI BANANA MUFFINS 207

GLUTEN-FREE PANCAKES 208

CINNAMON WAFFLES 209

CHEESE GRIT MUFFINS 210

CHOCHOLATE OATMEAL 212

DESSERTS 213

SPRINGTIME AVOCADO 213

APPLE YOGURT PARFAIT 214

YOGURT POPS 215

CHOCOLATE CHEESECAKES 216

LUSCIOUS LEMON PARFAIT 217

PUMPKIN CARAMEL CAKE 218

BLACK BEAN BROWNIES 219

BLUEBERRY BITES 221

APPLE PIE COOKIES 222

RICE BARS 223

SMOOTHIES 225

- BANANA SMOOTHIE 225
- LIVER DETOX SMOOTHIE 226
- GREEN PROTEIN SMOOTHIE 227
- CITRUS LIVER BOOST SMOOTHIE 228
- LIVER GREEN SMOOTHIE 229
- ARTICHOKE SMOOTHIE 230
- KALE LIVER DETOX SMOOTHIE 231
- ZUCCHINI LIVER DETOX SMOOTHIE 232
- SPRING LIVER DETOX SMOOTHIE 233
- STRAWBERRY MORNING SMOOTHIE 234
- LIVER ENERGY BOOSTING SMOOTHIE 235
- PAPAYA LIVER SMOOTHIE 236
- LIVER BLUEBERRIES SMOOTHIE 237
- TURMERIC LIVER SMOOTHIE 238
- BEETROOT LIVER DETOX SMOOTHIE 239
- CARROT & BEETROOT SMOOTHIE 240
- SPINACH LIVER DETOX SMOOTHIE 241
- APPLE CIDER SMOOTHIE 242
- GRAPEFRUIT SMOOTHIE 243
- KIWI SMOOTHIE 244

Copyright 2019 by Noah Jerris - All rights reserved.

This document is geared towards providing exact and reliable information in regards to the topic and issue covered. The publication is sold with the idea that the publisher is not required to render accounting, officially permitted, or otherwise, qualified services. If advice is necessary, legal or professional, a practiced individual in the profession should be ordered.

- From a Declaration of Principles which was accepted and approved equally by a Committee of the American Bar Association and a Committee of Publishers and Associations.

In no way is it legal to reproduce, duplicate, or transmit any part of this document in either electronic means or in printed format. Recording of this publication is strictly prohibited and any storage of this document is not allowed unless with written permission from the publisher. All rights reserved.

The information provided herein is stated to be truthful and consistent, in that any liability, in terms of inattention or otherwise, by any usage or abuse of any policies, processes, or directions contained within is the solitary and utter responsibility of the recipient reader. Under no circumstances will any legal responsibility or blame be held against the publisher for any reparation, damages, or monetary loss due to the information herein, either directly or indirectly.

Respective authors own all copyrights not held by the publisher.

The information herein is offered for informational purposes solely, and is universal as so. The presentation of the information is without contract or any type of guarantee assurance.

The trademarks that are used are without any consent, and the publication of the trademark is without permission or backing by the trademark owner. All trademarks and brands within this book are for clarifying purposes only and are the owned by the owners themselves, not affiliated with this document.

Introduction

Fatty liver recipes for personal enjoyment but also for family enjoyment. You will love them for sure for how easy it is to prepare them.

BREAKFAST

SKINNY OMELETTE

Serves: **2**

Prep Time: **10** Minutes

Cook Time: **10** Minutes

Total Time: **20** Minutes

INGREDIENTS

- 2 eggs
- pinch of salt
- 1 tablespoon chives
- 1 tablespoon pesto
- bit of goat cheese
- handful of salad greens

DIRECTIONS

1. In a bowl beat eggs and pour in a skillet over medium heat, sprinkle with chives, and spread the pesto across the omelette
2. Sprinkle salad greens, cheese and season with salt

VEGGIE QUINOA CUPS

Serves: **6**

Prep Time: **10** Minutes

Cook Time: **10** Minutes

Total Time: **20** Minutes

INGREDIENTS

- ½ cup quinoa
- 1 tablespoon olive oil
- 1 onion
- 3 cups spinach leaves
- 1 garlic clove
- ¼ shallot
- salt
- ¼ cup cheddar cheese
- ¼ cup parmesan cheese
- 1 egg

DIRECTIONS

1. Preheat oven to 350 F and line a six-cup muffin pan

2. Combine water and quinoa in a saucepan and bring to boil
3. Lower the heat and cook for 12-15 minutes, remove from heat and allow to cool
4. In a skillet heat oil, add onion and cook for 4-5 minutes
5. Stir in shallot, garlic and spinach and season with salt and pepper
6. Remove the pan from heat and mix with quinoa, pour in the eggs
7. Divide the batter into muffin cups and bake for 30-35 minutes

CRANBERRY STUFFING

Serves: 4
Prep Time: 10 Minutes
Cook Time: 10 Minutes
Total Time: 20 Minutes

INGREDIENTS

- 10 cups
- ½ cup butter
- 1 cup diced celery
- ¼ cup onion
- 1 cup chopped cranberries
- ½ cup sugar
- 1 tsp sage
- 1 tsp rosemary
- 1 tsp sage
- 1 tsp rosemary
- 1 tsp thyme
- ½ cup parsley
- salt
- 1 lb. ground sausage
- 1 cup chicken broth

DIRECTIONS

1. In a saucepan heat butter over medium heat, add onion, celery and cook, add cranberries, sage, sugar, rosemary, parsley, thyme
2. Season with salt and pepper
3. Brown the sausage in a skillet, drain off fat
4. Toss the ingredients in the bowl and add chicken broth
5. Serve when ready

CRUSTLESS QUICHE CUPS

Serves: **6**

Prep Time: **10** Minutes

Cook Time: **10** Minutes

Total Time: **20** Minutes

INGREDIENTS

- 10 oz. chopped kale
- 2 eggs
- 2 egg whites
- ½ cup leek
- ½ cup chopped tomato
- ½ cup bell pepper

DIRECTIONS

1. Preheat oven to 325 F and line a muffin pan with paper liners
2. In a bowl leek, egg whites, tomatoes, kale, eggs and bell pepper
3. Divide mixture into muffin cups and bake for 15-20 minutes
4. Remove and serve

QUINOA WITH SCALLIONS

Serves: **6**

Prep Time: **10** Minutes

Cook Time: **10** Minutes

Total Time: **20** Minutes

INGREDIENTS

- 3 ears corn
- 1 tablespoon lemon zest
- 1 tablespoon lemon juice
- ½ cup butter
- 1 tablespoon honey
- ¼ tsp salt
- ½ tsp pepper
- 1 cup quinoa
- 3 scallions

DIRECTIONS

1. In a pot place the corn and fill the pan with water, bring to boil and cover for 5-6 minutes
2. Remove from pot and let it cool

3. In a bowl mix the rest of the ingredients for dressing: lemon juice, melted butter, lemon zest, honey, pepper
4. Cook the quinoa in a pot, add scallions in a bowl with the dressing and toss well
5. Season with salt and serve

CORNBREAD MUFFINS

Serves: **4**
Prep Time: **10** Minutes

Cook Time: **20** Minutes

Total Time: **30** Minutes

INGREDIENTS

- 1 cup whole-wheat flour
- 1 can of Whole Kernel Corn 15 oz.
- ½ cup milk
- 1 egg
- ½ cup butter

- 1 tablespoon honey
- 1 tablespoon baking powder
- 1 tsp salt

DIRECTIONS

1. Preheat oven to 375 F
2. Blend corn until smooth
3. In a bowl mix baking powder, salt and flour
4. In another bowl mix eggs, butter, corn, milk and honey
5. Pour over the flour mixture and mix well
6. Pour mixture into a cupcake pan and bake for 15-20 minutes
7. Remove and serve

BERRY GRANOLA

Serves: **4**

Prep Time: **10** Minutes

Cook Time: **10** Minutes

Total Time: **20** Minutes

INGREDIENTS

- 2 tablespoons chia
- ¾ cup rolled oats
- 1 cup vanilla cashewmilk
- ½ cup fresh blueberries
- 2 strawberries
- ½ raspberries
- sprinkle of granola

DIRECTIONS

1. In a bowl mix cashewmilk, oats, chia and divide into 2 servings
2. Refrigerate overnight, remove top with berries and serve

OVERNIGHT OATS

Serves: 2

Prep Time: 5   Minutes

Cook Time: 5   Minutes

Total Time: 10 Minutes

INGREDIENTS

- 2 tablespoons chia
- ¾ cup rolled oats
- 1 cup vanilla cashewmilk
- ¼ cup peach
- ¼ plum
- 3 basil leaves
- 1 tsp pumpkin seeds
- 1 tsp hemp seeds

DIRECTIONS

1. In a bowl mix cashewmilk, oats, chia and oats, divide into 2-3 servings
2. Refrigerate overnight
3. Remove and serve

TROPICAL OVERNIGHT OATS

Serves: **4**

Prep Time: **10** Minutes

Cook Time: **20** Minutes

Total Time: **30** Minutes

INGREDIENTS

- 2 tablespoons chia
- ½ cup mango
- 1 banana
- ¼ avocado
- 1 tsp lemon juice
- 2/4 cup oats
- 1 cup vanilla Cashewmilk

DIRECTIONS

1. Mix oats, cashewmilk and chia seeds, divide into 2-3 servings
2. Refrigerate overnight
3. In a blender add lemon juice, banana, avocado and blend until smooth, top over oat mixture and serve

DETOX GREEN MORNING SMOOTHIE

Serves: 2
Prep Time: 5 Minutes
Cook Time: 5 Minutes
Total Time: 10 Minutes

INGREDIENTS

- 1 banana
- 1 tablespoon spirulina powder
- 1 green apple
- ¼ cup lime juice
- 1 cup spinach leaves
- 1 cucumber
- ¼ cup almond milk

DIRECTIONS

1. **In a blender place all ingredients and blend until smooth**
2. **Pour in a glass and serve**

BERRY DETOX PORRIDGE

Serves: *4*

Prep Time: *10* Minutes

Cook Time: *10* Minutes

Total Time: *20* Minutes

INGREDIENTS

- 1 cup oats
- 1 cup almond milk
- 1 tsp coconut oil
- 1 cup berries
- 2 tsp organic honey
- mixed seeds and nuts

DIRECTIONS

1. In a saucepan add milk, oats and bring to boil for 5-6 minutes
2. Transfer to a blender and blend until smooth
3. Pour into a bowl, add honey, berries and mixed seeds

MORNING COOKIES

Serves: *6*

Prep Time: *10* Minutes

Cook Time: *15* Minutes

Total Time: *25* Minutes

INGREDIENTS

- 3 bananas
- ¼ cup peanut butter
- ¼ cup cocoa powder
- handful of salt

DIRECTIONS

1. **Preheat oven to 325 F**
2. **In a bowl mix all ingredients**
3. **Form small cookies and place them onto a greased cookie sheet**
4. **Sprinkle with salt and bake for 12-15 minutes**
5. **Remove and serve**

AVOCADO AND EGG TOAST

Serves: 2

Prep Time: 5 Minutes

Cook Time: 5 Minutes

Total Time: 10 Minutes

INGREDIENTS

- 2 eggs
- 1 avocado
- 2 tsp tahini
- 2 tsp pumpkin seeds
- 2 tsp chia seeds
- 2 tablespoons tapenade
- black pepper
- 2-4 slices gluten-free toast

DIRECTIONS

1. Place avocado slices over toast and top with fried eggs
2. Add 1-2 tablespoons of tapenade paste on top of the toast and garnish with pumpkin and chia seeds

BREAFAST GLUTEN-FREE MUESLI

Serves: **4**

Prep Time: **5** Minutes

Cook Time: **5** Minutes

Total Time: **10** Minutes

INGREDIENTS

- 2 cups mixed seeds
- ¼ cup mixed dried fruit
- ¼ cup coconut flakes
- ¼ cup berries
- 1 banana
- non-dairy milk

DIRECTIONS

1. In a bowl add all dry ingredients and mix well
2. Refrigerate overnight
3. Remove and top with berries, banana, milk and serve

SWEET POTATO BREAKFAST WITH AVOCADO

Serves: *4*
Prep Time: *10* Minutes
Cook Time: *50* Minutes
Total Time: *60* Minutes

INGREDIENTS

- 1 sweet potato
- 1 tablespoon olive oil
- 2 cloves garlic
- 1 oz. beet greens
- 4 oz. baby spinach
- 5 eggs
- 1 avocado
- salt

DIRECTIONS

1. **Preheat oven to 375**
2. **Bake sweet potatoes for 55-60 minutes or until soft, remove potatoes and let them cook**

3. In a skillet heat oil over medium heat, add garlic, greens, spinach and sauté for 2-3 minutes
4. Divide between 2 bowls, add sweet potatoes, avocado, eggs and serve

MORNING BLACKBERRY COCONUT BOWL

Serves: *4*

Prep Time: *10* Minutes

Cook Time: *10* Minutes

Total Time: *20* Minutes

INGREDIENTS

- 1 cup blackberries
- 1 banana
- ½ cup coconut flakes
- 1 cup coconut milk
- 1 tsp chia seeds
- 1 tsp pumpkin seeds
- ¼ cup spinach

DIRECTIONS

1. In a blender add milk, spinach, banana and blend until smooth
2. Add berries and distribute mixture into a serving bowl
3. Top with pumpkin seeds, coconut flakes and serve

COCONUT YOGURT WITH BERRIES

Serves: **4**

Prep Time: **10** Minutes

Cook Time: **10** Minutes

Total Time: **20** Minutes

INGREDIENTS

- 1 cup coconut milk
- 1 tablespoon sunflower seeds
- 1 tablespoon shredded coconut
- pinch of cinnamon

- ½ cup berries
- 1 tsp stevia

DIRECTIONS

1. In a bowl add yogurt and coconut milk
2. Top with cinnamon, coconut, sunflower seeds and berries
3. Add stevia and serve

RASPBERRY SORBET

Serves: **4**
Prep Time: **10** Minutes

Cook Time: **10** Minutes

Total Time: **20** Minutes

INGREDIENTS

- 1 cup raspberries
- ½ cup sugar

- 2 cups water
- 1 cup orange juice
- ½ cup agave syrup
- ¼ cup apple cider vinegar

DIRECTIONS

1. In a pot mix all ingredients over high meat, bring to boil for 8-10 minutes
2. Transfer to a blender and blend until smooth
3. Pour into a bowl and serve

AVOCADO BROWNIE

Serves: *4*

Prep Time: *10* Minutes

Cook Time: *30* Minutes

Total Time: *40* Minutes

INGREDIENTS

- 1 ripe avocado
- 3 tablespoons melted butter
- 1 egg
- ¼ cup brown sugar
- ¼ maple syrup
- 1 tablespoon vanilla extract
- ¾ cup cocoa powder
- ½ tsp salt
- ½ cup gluten-free flour
- ¼ cup dark chocolate chips

DIRECTIONS

1. Preheat the oven to 325 F
2. In a bowl mash the avocado, brown sugar, maple syrup, vanilla, sugar, water, butter, add cocoa powder
3. In a bowl mix salt and flour and stir in avocado mixture, spread bake in the pan and bake for 35 minutes
4. Remove and cool before serving

BANANA PANCAKES

Serves: **4**

Prep Time: **10** Minutes

Cook Time: **10** Minutes

Total Time: **20** Minutes

INGREDIENTS

- 1 banana
- 2 eggs
- 1,2 oz. flour
- 1 cup honey

DIRECTIONS

1. **In a bowl mix all ingredients except honey**
2. **Pour pancake mixture into a skillet and cook for 1-2 minutes per side**
3. **Remove pancakes onto a plate and serve with honey**

LUNCH

MINESTRONE SOUP

Serves: **6**

Prep Time: **10** Minutes

Cook Time: **50** Minutes

Total Time: **60** Minutes

INGREDIENTS

- 2 onions
- 1 cup peas
- 1 can tomatoes
- 2 cups tomato sauce
- 3 carrots
- 1 cup green beans
- 2 tbs basil
- 6 cups water
- 2 cloves garlic
- Salt
- 2 tbs cheese
- 1.5 cups kidney
- 2 cups celery

- 1 bell pepper

DIRECTIONS

1. Put the onions, celery and carrots into a pot of water.
2. Add the green beans, peas, tomatoes and bell pepper when the water starts to boil, then allow to boil for 30 minutes.
3. Add the tomato sauce and basil then season with salt.
4. Allow to simmer for 10 minutes, then add the garlic and simmer for 5 more minutes.
5. Serve topped with cheese.

TUNA SALAD

Serves.   *4*
Prep Time: *10*   Minutes
Cook Time: *5*   Minutes
Total Time: *15*   Minutes

INGREDIENTS
- ½ tsp lemon zest
- Salt
- Pepper
- 4 eggs
- 1/3 red onion
- ¾ lb green beans
- 1 can tuna
- 1 tsp oregano
- 6 tbs olive oil
- 3 tbs lemon juice
- 1 can beans
- 1 can black olives

DIRECTIONS

1. Place the green beans, 1/3 cup water and salt to taste in a skillet.
2. Bring to a boil, covered.
3. Cook for 5 minutes.
4. Dump them onto a lined cookie sheet.
5. Mix the white beans, onion, olives and tuna.
6. Combine the oregano, lemon juice and zest, and oil in a separate bowl.
7. Pour the mixture over the tuna mixture.
8. Season and serve immediately with the boiled eggs.

CHICKEN SKILLET

Serves: **4**

Prep Time: **10** Minutes

Cook Time: **30** Minutes

Total Time: **40** Minutes

INGREDIENTS

- 1 tsp oil
- ½ cup carrots
- 1 zucchini
- 1 bell pepper
- ½ lb chicken
- 1 onion

DIRECTIONS

1. Cut the chicken into strips, then cook in the oil until it gets brown.
2. Remove from the skillet and add the vegetables.
3. Cook until soft for 10 minutes, then add the chicken.
4. Season and serve immediately.

SPINACH QUESADILLAS

Serves: **4**

Prep Time: **10** Minutes

Cook Time: **15** Minutes

Total Time: **25** Minutes

INGREDIENTS

- 4 cups spinach
- 4 green onions
- 1 tomato
- ½ lemon juice
- 1 tsp cumin
- 1 tsp garlic powder
- Salt
- 1 cup cheese
- 4 tortillas

DIRECTIONS

1. Cook all of the ingredients except for the cheese and tortillas in a skillet.
2. Cook until the spinach is wilted.

3. Remove to a bowl and add the cheese.
4. Place the mixture on half of the tortilla, fold the other half and cook for 2 minutes on each side on a griddle.
5. Serve immediately.

BEAN SALAD

Serves: **4**

Prep Time: **10** Minutes

Cook Time: **0** Minutes

Total Time: **10** Minutes

INGREDIENTS

- 1 can garbanzo beans
- 1 can red beans
- 1 tomato
- ½ red onion
- ½ lemon juice
- 1 tbs olive oil

DIRECTIONS

1. Mix all of the ingredients together in a bowl.
2. Season with salt and serve immediately.

GARLIC SALMON

Serves: **4**

Prep Time: **10** Minutes

Cook Time: **20** Minutes

Total Time: **30** Minutes

INGREDIENTS

- 2 lb salmon
- 2 tbs water
- Salt
- 2 tbs parsley
- 4 cloves garlic

DIRECTIONS

1. Preheat the oven to 400F.
2. Mix the garlic, parsley, salt and water in a bowl.
3. Brush the mixture over the salmon.
4. Place the fish on a baking tray and cover with aluminum foil.
5. Cook for 20 minutes.
6. Serve with vegetables.

TUNA WRAP

Serves: **4**

Prep Time: **10** Minutes

Cook Time: **0** Minutes

Total Time: **10** Minutes

INGREDIENTS

- 6 ounces tuna
- 2 tsp yogurt

- ½ celery stalk
- Handful baby spinach
- ½ onion
- 2 tsp lemon juice
- 4 tortillas

DIRECTIONS

1. Mix all of the ingredients except for the tortillas in a bowl.
2. Spread the mixture over the tortillas, then wrap them up.
3. Serve immediately.

ROASTED CHICKEN WRAP

Serves: *4*
Prep Time: *10* Minutes
Cook Time: *10* Minutes
Total Time: *20* Minutes

INGREDIENTS

- 1 cup chicken breast
- 2 tsp yogurt
- 1/3 cup celery
- 8 tomato slices
- ½ onion
- 1 tbs mustard
- 2 tbs ketchup
- 4 tortillas

DIRECTIONS

1. Cut the chicken as you desire and grill until done on each side.
2. Mix all of the ingredients except for the tortillas in a bowl.
3. Spread the mixture over the tortillas and add the chicken.
4. Serve immediately.

LENTIL SALAD

Serves: **4**

Prep Time: **10** Minutes

Cook Time: **0** Minutes

Total Time: **10** Minutes

INGREDIENTS

- 1 cup cooked lentils
- 1 cup baby spinach
- 1 poached egg
- ¼ avocado
- ½ tomato
- 1-2 slices whole wheat bread

DIRECTIONS

1. **Mix all of the ingredients together except for the bread.**
2. **Toast the bread.**
3. **Serve immediately together.**

STUFFED EGGPLANT

Serves: **4**

Prep Time: **10** Minutes

Cook Time: **50** Minutes

Total Time: **60** Minutes

INGREDIENTS
- 1 eggplant
- 2 onions
- 1 red pepper
- ½ cup tomato juice
- ¼ cup cheese

DIRECTIONS

1. Preheat the oven to 350F.
2. Cut the eggplant in half and cook for 30 minutes.
3. Cook the diced onion in 2 tbs of water until brown.
4. Add the pepper and add it to the onion, cooking for another 5 minutes.
5. Add the tomato juice and allow to cook for another 5 minutes.
6. Scoop out the eggplant.

7. Mix the eggplant with the onion mixture, then add it back into the eggplant shell.
8. Grate the cheese on top and bake for another 10 minutes.
9. Serve hot.

BROCCOLI & AURGULA SOUP

Serves: 2
Prep Time: 5 Minutes
Cook Time: 20 Minutes
Total Time: 25 Minutes

INGREDIENTS

- 1 tbs olive oil
- ¼ tsp thyme
- 1 cup arugula
- ½ lemon juice
- 1 head broccoli
- 1 clove garlic

- 2 cups water
- ¼ tsp salt
- ¼ tsp black pepper
- ½ yellow onion

DIRECTIONS

1. Heat the oil in a saucepan.
2. Cook the onion until soft, then add the garlic and cook for another minute.
3. Add the broccoli and cook for 5 minutes.
4. Add the water, thyme, salt, and pepper.
5. Bring to boil, then lower the heat and cook for 10 minutes.
6. Transfer to a blender, blend, then add the arugula and blend until smooth.
7. Add the lemon juice and serve immediately.

STUFFED PEPPERS

Serves: **4**

Prep Time: **20** Minutes

Cook Time: **25** Minutes

Total Time: **45** Minutes

INGREDIENTS

- ½ onion
- 1 cup mushrooms
- ½ yellow bell pepper
- 1 cup spinach
- 1 can tomatoes
- 1 tbs tomato paste
- 4 red bell peppers
- 1 lb ground turkey
- 2 tbs olive oil
- 1 zucchini
- ½ green bell pepper
- 1 tsp Italian seasoning
- ½ tsp garlic powder
- Salt
- Pepper

DIRECTIONS

1. Bring a pot of water to a boil.
2. Cut the tops off the peppers, and remove the seeds.
3. Cook in water for 5 minutes.
4. Preheat the oven to 350F.
5. Cook the turkey until brown.
6. Heat the oil and cook the onion, mushrooms, zucchini, green and yellow pepper, and spinach until soft.
7. Add the turkey and the rest of the ingredients.
8. Stuff the peppers with the mixture.
9. Bake for 15 minutes.

POTATO SALAD

Serves: 6
Prep Time: 5 Minutes
Cook Time: 10 Minutes
Total Time: 15 Minutes

INGREDIENTS

- 1 red onion
- 2 tsp cumin seeds
- 1 cloves garlic
- ½ cup olive oil
- 4 potatoes
- ½ cup lemon juice
- 2 tbs fresh parsley
- 1 ½ tsp salt
- 2 tsp turmeric powder

DIRECTIONS

1. Steam the potatoes for 10 minutes, until tender.
2. Mix the lemon juice, turmeric, cumin seeds, and salt.
3. Place the potatoes in a bowl and pour the mixture over.
4. Add the onion and garlic and stir to coat.
5. Refrigerate until the potatoes are cold.
6. Add olive oil and herbs and stir.

PORK TACOS

Serves: **4**

Prep Time: **20** Minutes

Cook Time: **10** Minutes

Total Time: **30** Minutes

INGREDIENTS

- 1 cucumber
- 1 cup red cabbage
- 1 ½ lbs ground pork
- 6 radishes
- 4 tsp sugar
- 2 tbs olive oil
- ¼ cup white wine vinegar
- 2 tbs soy sauce
- 2 tsp garlic powder
- 2 tbs sesame oil
- 4 scallions
- 2 tsp Sriracha
- 12 tortillas
- 2 tsp cilantro
- ½ cup sour cream

- Salt
- Pepper

DIRECTIONS

1. Place the cucumbers, radishes, vinegar, 2 tsp sugar, salt, and pepper in a bowl.
2. Cook the scallions and cabbage in the oil until soft.
3. Add the pork, garlic powder, and 2 tsp sugar and cook for another 5 minutes.
4. Add the sesame oil, Sriracha, soy sauce and combine.
5. Season with salt and pepper.
6. Heat the tortillas in the microwave for a few seconds.
7. Spread sour cream on the tortilla, add the mixture, sprinkle cilantro over and add the cucumber and radishes.
8. Serve immediately.

CHICKEN & AVOCADO SALAD

Serves: **4**

Prep Time: **15** Minutes

Cook Time: **5** Minutes

Total Time: **20** Minutes

INGREDIENTS

- 1 avocado
- ½ cup celery
- ¼ cup red onion
- 2 tbs cilantro
- 1 apple
- 2 tsp lime juice
- 1 chicken breast
- Salt
- Pepper
- Olive oil

DIRECTIONS

1. Slice the chicken and season with salt and pepper.
2. Cook the chicken in a skillet until done.

3. Allow to cool for a few minutes, then dice and place in a bowl.
4. Dice the veggies and place in the chicken bowl.
5. Mix well the ingredients.
6. Sprinkle in the cilantro.
7. Add lime juice and season with salt and pepper.
8. Serve on a bed of greens.

PHILLY CHEESE STEAK

Serves: 4
Prep Time: 5 Minutes
Cook Time: 20 Minutes
Total Time: 25 Minutes

INGREDIENTS

- 2 tsp olive oil
- 1 onion
- 3 ounces cheese
- 4 whole-wheat rolls

- 2 tsp oregano
- ½ tsp ground pepper
- 1 tbs flour
- ¼ cup vegetable broth
- 1 red bell pepper
- 4 mushrooms
- 1 tbs soy sauce

DIRECTIONS

1. Cook the onion in the oil for 5 minutes, until soft.
2. Add the mushrooms, bell pepper, oregano and pepper and cook until soft.
3. Reduce the heap and sprinkle with flour, stirring to coat.
4. Stir in the soy sauce and bring to a boil.
5. Place the cheese slices over the vegetables, cover and allow to melt.
6. Split and toast the rolls, spread the mixture into the rolls and serve

MAPLE-ROASTED SWEET POTATOES

Serves: **15**

Prep Time: **15** Minutes

Cook Time: **60** Minutes

Total Time: **75** Minutes

INGREDIENTS

- 1 tbs lemon juice
- ½ tsp salt
- 2 tbs butter
- 2 ½ lb sweet potatoes
- 1/3 cup maple syrup
- 1 red onion

DIRECTIONS

1. Preheat the oven to 400F.
2. Mix the maple syrup, lemon juice, butter, salt and pepper in a bowl.
3. Peel and cut the potatoes into cubes.
4. Place them on a baking dish and pour the maple syrup mixture over, then toss to coat.

5. Cover with foil and cook for 15 minutes, then cook uncovered for 1 hour, stirring frequently.
6. Serve immediately.

MUSHROOM SOUP

Serves: *4*

Prep Time: *10* Minutes

Cook Time: *30* Minutes

Total Time: *40* Minutes

INGREDIENTS

- 2 onions
- 40 ounces mushrooms
- 1 tbs soy sauce
- 20 stalks fresh thyme
- 2 tbs flour
- 2 cups vegetable broth
- 2 cups almond milk
- Pepper

- 2 bay leaves

DIRECTIONS

1. Sweat the onions for 5 minutes in a saucepan.
2. Add the mushrooms in the center of the saucepan and cook for another 5 minutes.
3. Stir the onions and mushrooms together, add the thyme and cook for at least 10 minutes.
4. Add the bay leaf, salt and soy sauce.
5. Stir the flour into the vegetable broth in a bowl, then add it to the mushrooms.
6. Add the almond milk to the pan.
7. Allow to cook for 15 minutes, then season with the pepper, serve immediately.

DETOX SALAD

Serves: 4
Prep Time: 30   Minutes
Cook Time: 0   Minutes
Total Time: 30   Minutes

INGREDIENTS

Salad:
- ½ head of red cabbage
- 2 tbs flax seed
- 2 tbs sunflower seeds
- 2 celery sticks
- 3 tbs pine nuts
- 2 apples
- 3 carrots
- 2 tbs parsley
- 1 tbs pumpkin seeds

Dressing:
- 4 tbs olive oil
- 1 tsp honey
- 2 tsp ginger root
- 2 tbs lemon juice

DIRECTIONS

1. Mix all of the ingredients together.
2. Whisk the dressing ingredients in a bowl.
3. Pour the dressing over and toss to coat.
4. Serve immediately.

ROASTED ASPARAGUS

Serves: **8**

Prep Time: **10** Minutes

Cook Time: **30** Minutes

Total Time: **40** Minutes

INGREDIENTS

- 2 lb asparagus
- 1 tsp thyme leaves
- 2 tsp olive oil
- Salt
- ½ lemon juice
- 1 tbs lemon zest
- Black pepper

DIRECTIONS

1. Preheat the oven to 400F.
2. Break off the ends of the asparagus.
3. Place it on a baking sheet, drizzle with olive oil and toss to coat.
4. Season with salt and pepper.

5. Roast for 30 minutes.
6. Remove from oven and sprinkle with thyme.
7. Drizzle on lemon juice and sprinkle with zest.
8. Serve immediately.

DINNER

GARLICKY TOFU

Serves: **4**

Prep Time: **10** Minutes

Cook Time: **10** Minutes

Total Time: **20** Minutes

INGREDIENTS

- 2 tablespoons olive oil
- 2 tablespoons crushed garlic
- salt
- 12-oz. tofu
- black pepper

DIRECTIONS

1. Cut tofu in 1-inch cubes and place in a bowl with olive oil, pepper and garlic
2. In a pan add the tofu mixture and sauté for 5-6 minutes
3. Remove and serve

PORK MEATBALLS

Serves: *4*
Prep Time: *20* Minutes
Cook Time: *30* Minutes
Total Time: *50* Minutes

INGREDIENTS

- 4 tablespoons olive oil
- 1 egg
- ½ tsp cumin
- ½ tsp turmeric

- ¼ tsp paprika
- salt
- 1 onion
- ¼ cup fresh parsley leaves
- 1 tablespoons Worcestershire sauce
- 2 lbs. fatty ground beef
- ¼ lb. duck
- ¼ cup bread crumbs

DIRECTIONS

1. In a skillet heat oil over medium heat, add onions sauté for 2-3 minutes, transfer to a bowl and add parsley and Worcestershire sauce
2. Add ground beef, livers, eggs, paprika, turmeric, cumin and mix well, add salt and pepper
3. Preheat oven to 400, place the meatballs on a baking sheet
4. Bake for 15-20 minutes, garnish with cheese and serve

ITALIAN PATE WITH FRIED ANCHOVIES

Serves: **10**

Prep Time: **10** Minutes

Cook Time: **30** Minutes

Total Time: **40** Minutes

INGREDIENTS

- 1 ½ lb. chicken liver
- ½ cup avocado oil
- 2 shallots
- 1 garlic clove
- 1 oz. anchovy fillet
- ½ cup capers
- 1 tsp ground sage
- 1 tsp lemon zest
- 1 tablespoon lemon juice

DIRECTIONS

1. Trim your chicken livers and any piece of fat
2. Place the trimmed chicken livers into a bowl, smash cloves

3. Drain the anchovy fillets
4. In a skillet add oil, garlic, shallots, anchovy fillets and capers
5. Cook until golden brown and sprinkle with sage
6. Remove skillet from heat and transfer to a blender, add lemon zest, lemon juice
7. Taste and pour pate into a dish

VEGETABLE FRITTATA

Serves: **4**

Prep Time: **15** Minutes

Cook Time: **20** Minutes

Total Time: **35** Minutes

INGREDIENTS

- 2 egg
- 3 egg whites
- ½ cup parmesan cheese
- 1 tsp turmeric

- ¼ cup orange bell pepper
- ¼ cup red onion
- 1 tsp garlic
- ¼ tsp olive oil
- 1 cup spinach
- salt

DIRECTIONS

1. Whisk the egg whites and eggs in a bowl
2. Add garlic, bell pepper, red onion, parmesan, turmeric and mix well
3. In a pan add egg mixture and spinach leaves
4. Season with salt and pepper and serve

CHICKEN LIVER PATE

Serves: **4**

Prep Time: **10** Minutes

Cook Time: **15** Minutes

Total Time: **25** Minutes

INGREDIENTS

- 1 lb. chicken livers
- ¼ lb. butter
- 1 tablespoons brandy
- 2 tablespoons heavy cream
- 1 orange zest

DIRECTIONS

1. Remove the fat and cut each liver in half
2. In a saucepan melt butter, add chicken livers and cook for 10-12 minutes
3. Remove from heat add brandy, orange zest, orange juice and cream
4. Puree until smooth and season with salt
5. Pour into ramekin dishes and serve

LAMB LIBERS WITH KALE AND LEMON

Serves: **4**

Prep Time: **10** Minutes

Cook Time: **15** Minutes

Total Time: **25** Minutes

INGREDIENTS

- 1 lb. chicken livers
- 1 tsp oil
- ¼ salt
- ¼ tsp pepper
- 4 green onions
- 1 cup kale pieces
- 1 cup water
- ½ cup lemon juice

DIRECTIONS

1. In a skillet heat oil over medium heat and add chicken livers and sprinkle with salt
2. Cook for 5-10 minutes
3. Remove and to a plate

4. In the skillet add kale, water and green onions, bring to boil
5. Slice the livers, return to the skillet and add lemon juice, serve when ready

DANISH LIVER PATE

Serves: **4**

Prep Time: **10** Minutes

Cook Time: **50** Minutes

Total Time: **60** Minutes

INGREDIENTS

- 1 lb. liver
- 2/3 lb. bacon bits
- 1 tsp salt
- 1 tsp pepper
- 1 egg
- 1 tablespoon flour
- 4 oz. milk

DIRECTIONS

1. Preheat oven to 200 F
2. In a blender add bacon, onion and liver and blend until smooth
3. Add the rest of the ingredients and mix well
4. Pour mixture into a greased loaf pan
5. Bake for 50-60 minutes
6. Remove and serve

CHICKEN SALSA

Serves: **4**

Prep Time: **10** Minutes

Cook Time: **20** Minutes

Total Time: **30** Minutes

INGREDIENTS

- 1 lb. chicken breast

- 1 onion
- 1 red pepper
- 1 tomato
- 1 can kidney beans
- 2 cloves garlic
- 1 cup salsa
- 1 bunch broccoli
- cilantro
- olive oil
- salt

DIRECTIONS

1. In a skillet sauté garlic, onion, add pepper and cook for 2-3 minutes
2. Add pepper, bring mixture to boil
3. Reduce the heat and simmer 5-6 minutes
4. Remove and serve with chicken

SPAGHETTI SQUASH HASH BROWNS

Serves: **4**

Prep Time: **10** Minutes

Cook Time: **15** Minutes

Total Time: **25** Minutes

INGREDIENTS

- 2 cups shredded squash
- 1 tablespoon oil

DIRECTIONS

1. In a skillet heat oil over medium heat
2. Remove water out of the squash
3. Place the patties on the skillet and cook for 6-7 minutes
4. Remove and transfer to a paper towel

BAKED PAPRIKA CHICKEN

Serves: **4**

Prep Time: **10** Minutes

Cook Time: **40** Minutes

Total Time: **50** Minutes

INGREDIENTS

- 2 lb. chicken pieces
- 2 lb. pumpkin
- 1 tablespoon paprika powder
- ½ cup pine nuts
- 1 spring rosemary
- 2 tablespoons olive oil
- salt

DIRECTIONS
1. Preheat oven to 375 F and place the chicken into an oven dish
2. Brush with olive oil and add pumpkin
3. Sprinkle salt, paprika, rosemary and bake for 25-30 minutes
4. Remove, add pine nuts and cook for another 5-10 minutes

CAULIFLOWER AND QUINOA SALAD

Serves: **4**

Prep Time: **10** Minutes

Cook Time: **30** Minutes

Total Time: **40** Minutes

INGREDIENTS

- ¼ head cauliflower
- 1 tablespoon olive oil
- ¼ tsp cumin
- 1 cup quinoa
- 1 handful parsley
- ½ cup pecans
- salt

DIRECTIONS

1. **Preheat oven to 400 F**
2. **Roast cauliflower in the oven until golden**
3. **In a bowl mix all salad ingredients and serve**

RASPBERRY BREAD

Serves: **6**

Prep Time: **10** Minutes

Cook Time: **40** Minutes

Total Time: **50** Minutes

INGREDIENTS

- 2 cups almond meal
- 2 tablespoons almond butter
- 2 eggs
- 1 tsp vanilla essence
- 1 cup raspberries
- ¼ cup pecan pieces

DIRECTIONS

1. Preheat oven to 325 F
2. In a bowl beat eggs and mix with almond butter
3. Add remaining ingredients
4. Spoon the mixture into a loaf pan and bake for 40 minutes
5. Remove and serve

GREEK LAMB MEATBALLS

Serves: **4**
Prep Time: **10** Minutes
Cook Time: **25** Minutes
Total Time: **40** Minutes

INGREDIENTS

- 1 lb. ground lamb
- 1 egg
- 1 cloves garlic
- 1 handful parsley
- 1 tablespoon dried oregano
- 1 tsp dried rosemary
- ½ cup fetta cheese
- ¼ tsp salt

DIRECTIONS

1. **Preheat the oven to 325 F**
2. **In a bowl mix all ingredients**
3. **Form into meat balls**
4. **Bake for 20-25 minutes, remove and serv**

BAKED CHILLI CHICKEN

Serves: **4**

Prep Time: **10** Minutes

Cook Time: **30** Minutes

Total Time: **40** Minutes

INGREDIENTS

- 2 lb. chicken drumsticks
- 3 tablespoons olive oil
- 2 cloves garlic
- 2 tablespoons lime juice
- 3 tsp lime zest
- 1 tsp chilli flakes
- salt

DIRECTIONS

1. In a bowl place all ingredients except chicken drumsticks
2. Refrigerate and then add the drumsticks for 1-2 hours
3. Preheat oven to 350 F

4. Arrange the chicken drumsticks on a greased oven tray and bake for 40-45 minutes
5. Remove and serve

BROCCOLI STIR FRY

Serves: 2

Prep Time: 10 Minutes

Cook Time: 15 Minutes

Total Time: 25 Minutes

INGREDIENTS

- 1 head broccoli
- 1 handful cashews
- 1 tablespoons macadamia nut oil
- 2 tablespoons coconut aminos
- 1 tablespoon fish sauce
- 2 cloves garlic
- ¼ red pepper
- 1 tablespoon lime juice

- 6 oz. shrimp
- 1 tablespoon sesame seeds
- salt

DIRECTIONS

1. In a frying pan heat oil over medium heat
2. Add garlic, sesame seeds, red pepper and cashews
3. Add shrimp and fry for 3-4 minutes
4. Remove and serve

EGGPLANT FRIES

Serves: *4*
Prep Time: *10* Minutes
Cook Time: *30* Minutes
Total Time: *40* Minutes

INGREDIENTS

- 1 eggplant

- 1 cup almond meal
- 1 tsp oregano
- 1 tsp cumin
- 1 tsp coriander
- ¼ tsp salt
- 1 egg
- 1 tablespoon olive oil

DIRECTIONS

1. Preheat oven to 425 F
2. Whisk the egg with olive oil
3. In another bowl mix herbs, salt, almond meal and spices
4. Dip eggplant into each bowl, first in egg mixture and then coat in the almond meal mixture
5. Bake for 20-25 minutes
6. Remove and serve

GLUTEN FREE BANANA CAKE

Serves: **4**

Prep Time: **10** Minutes

Cook Time: **55** Minutes

Total Time: **65** Minutes

INGREDIENTS

- 3 bananas
- 3 eggs
- ¼ cup peanut butter
- 3 tablespoons coconut oil
- ¼ cup almond meal
- ½ cup pecans
- 1 tsp cloves
- 1 tsp cinnamon
- 1 tsp baking soda
- 1 tsp baking powder

DIRECTIONS

1. **Preheat oven to 325 F**

2. In a bowl mix eggs, bananas, peanuts butter and place in a blender, blend until smooth
3. Pour mixture into a cake tin and bake for 50-60 minutes, remove and serve

SEAFOOD CURRY

Serves: *4*

Prep Time: *10* Minutes

Cook Time: *20* Minutes

Total Time: *30* Minutes

INGREDIENTS

- 1 lb. white fish
- 13 oz. coconut milk
- 1 cup vegetable stock
- 1 carrot
- 1 onion
- 1 cup pumpkin
- 1 zucchini
- 1 tablespoon curry powder

- 1 tsp garam masala
- 2 cloves garlic

DIRECTIONS

1. In a pot place all ingredients except fish
2. Bring mixture to boil, cook for 4-5 minutes
3. Remove and serve

MASHED SWEET POTATOES

Serves: **4**

Prep Time: **10** Minutes

Cook Time: **15** Minutes

Total Time: **25** Minutes

INGREDIENTS

- 2 lb. sweet potatoes
- 1 tablespoon olive oil
- ¼ onion

- 1 garlic clove
- 1 tsp oregano
- ½ cu Greek yogurt
- salt

DIRECTIONS

1. Sauté the onion for 4-5 minutes
2. Bake potatoes until soft
3. In a bowl mix all ingredients and add potatoes and mix well
4. Serve with seafood

GARLIC SPICY CHICKEN

Serves: 4
Prep Time: 10 Minutes
Cook Time: 20 Minutes
Total Time: 30 Minutes

INGREDIENTS

- 2 lb. chicken drumsticks
- 1 tablespoon garlic powder
- 1 tablespoon paprika
- 1 tablespoon cumin
- ¼ tsp chili powder
- ¼ tsp salt
- ½ cup olive oil

DIRECTIONS

1. In a bowl place all ingredients
2. Add chicken drumsticks and cook them with the mixture
3. Cook the chicken for 15-20 minutes or until golden brown, remove and serve

DESSERTS & SMOOTHIES

BLUEBERRY BITES

Serves: 8
Prep Time: 5 Minutes
Cook Time: 30 Minutes
Total Time: 35 Minutes

INGREDIENTS

- 2 cups oats
- ½ tsp cinnamon
- 1 cup blueberries
- ½ cup honey
- ½ cup almond butter
- 1 tsp vanilla

DIRECTIONS

1. Mix all of the ingredients together, except for the blueberries.

2. Fold in the blueberries and refrigerate for 30 minutes.
3. Form balls from the mixture and serve.

WATERMELON SMOOTHIE

Serves: 2
Prep Time: 5 Minutes
Cook Time: 0 Minutes
Total Time: 5 Minutes

INGREDIENTS

- 2 cups watermelon
- 2 cups pineapple
- 1 ½ cups coconut water
- 1 orange
- 1 tsp ginger
- 2 tsp turmeric
- 2 drops of stevia
- ½ cup coconut milk

DIRECTIONS

1. Blend all of the ingredients together until smooth.
2. Serve immediately.

GINGER LEMONADE

Serves: **8**

Prep Time: **5** Minutes

Cook Time: **10** Minutes

Total Time: **15** Minutes

INGREDIENTS

- 1/3 cup honey
- 4 lemons juice
- Ice
- 4 strips of lemon peel
- 2 tbs ginger root
- 2 sprigs rosemary

DIRECTIONS

1. Mix the honey, ginger, lemon peel and 2 sprigs rosemary in a pot with 2 cups water.
2. Bring to a boil, then simmer for 10 minutes.
3. Remove from heat and allow to cool for 15 minutes.
4. Strain into a pitcher.
5. Discard the ginger and rosemary.
6. Add 6 cups of cold water and lemon juice to the pitcher.
7. Stir to combine and serve with ice.

LIME GRILLED CORN

Serves: **4**

Prep Time: **5** Minutes

Cook Time: **15** Minutes

Total Time: **20** Minutes

INGREDIENTS

- 4 corns

- 2 tbs mayonnaise
- Salt
- Pepper
- 2 tbs lime juice
- ¼ tsp chili powder

DIRECTIONS

1. Preheat the grill.
2. Cook the shucked corn onto the grill for 5 minutes.
3. Turn every few minutes until all sides are charred.
4. Mix the mayonnaise, chili powder, and lime juice in a bowl.
5. Season with salt and pepper and add lime juice and chili powder.
6. Serve coated with the mayonnaise mixture.

MOCKTAIL

Serves: *1*

Prep Time: *10* Minutes

Cook Time: *0* Minutes

Total Time: *10* Minutes

INGREDIENTS

- Ice
- 6 ounces soda water
- 3 lime slices
- 11 mint leaves
- 1 tbs honey

DIRECTIONS

1. Add mint leaves and lime to a glass and muddle with a spoon.
2. Add honey, ice and soda.
3. Stir to combine.
4. Serve garnished with lime and mint.

BANANA MUFFINS

Serves: 8
Prep Time: 5 Minutes
Cook Time: 25 Minutes
Total Time: 30 Minutes

INGREDIENTS

- ½ cup oats
- 1 can white beans
- ¼ tsp salt
- ¼ cup peanut butter
- ¼ cup maple syrup
- ¾ tsp baking soda
- 2 tsp vanilla
- 1/8 baking soda
- 1 banana

DIRECTIONS

1. **Preheat the oven to 350F.**
2. **Line 8 muffin cups.**
3. **Blend all ingredients until smooth.**

4. Pour into the muffin cups and bake for 20 minutes.
5. Serve warm.

APPLE CRUMBLE

Serves: **6**

Prep Time: **10** Minutes

Cook Time: **30** Minutes

Total Time: **40** Minutes

INGREDIENTS

- 4 apples
- 2 tsp cinnamon
- 1 cup flour
- ½ cup walnuts
- 2 cups quinoa
- 1/3 cup ground almonds

DIRECTIONS

1. Preheat the oven to 350F.

2. Oil a baking dish.
3. Place the apples into prepared dishes.
4. Mix the remaining ingredients in a bowl.
5. Crumble over the apples.
6. Bake for 30 minutes.
7. Serve immediately.

GINGERSNAPS

Serves: *18*
Prep Time: *10* Minutes
Cook Time: *10* Minutes
Total Time: *20* Minutes

INGREDIENTS

- 1 ¾ cups flour
- 1 ¾ ground ginger
- ¼ tsp ground cinnamon
- 1/8 tsp nutmeg
- 1/8 tsp cloves

- 1 ½ tsp cornstarch
- ¼ cup milk
- ¼ cup molasses
- 3 tbs Swerve
- ¼ tsp salt
- 2 tbs butter
- 1 egg white
- 2 ¼ tsp vanilla
- 2 tsp stevia
- 1 tsp baking powder

DIRECTIONS

1. Preheat the oven to 325F.
2. Mix the cornstarch, nutmeg, flour, cloves, ginger, cinnamon, baking powder, and salt in a bowl.
3. In another bowl, whisk the butter, egg, vanilla, and stevia.
4. Stir in the molasses and milk.
5. Incorporate the flour mixture.
6. Divide into 18 portions and roll into balls.
7. Roll in the Swerve until coated.
8. Place on a lined baking sheet.
9. Sprinkle with Swerve and bake for 10 minutes.
10. Allow to cool, then serve.

RICE KRISPIES

Serves: **16**

Prep Time: **10** Minutes

Cook Time: **60** Minutes

Total Time: **70** Minutes

INGREDIENTS

- 4 cups rice cereal
- 2 tbs dark chocolate
- 2/3 cup honey
- ½ cup peanut butter
- Salt
- 1 tsp vanilla

DIRECTIONS

1. Combine all of the ingredients except for the dark chocolate in a bowl.
2. Spread the mixture on a lined baking pan.
3. Drizzle the melted chocolate on top.
4. Refrigerate for 1 hour.
5. Cut into bars and serve.

APPLE OATMEAL COOKIES

Serves: **15**

Prep Time: **40** Minutes

Cook Time: **15** Minutes

Total Time: **55** Minutes

INGREDIENTS

- 1 cup oats
- ¾ cup flour
- 1 tsp vanilla
- ½ cup maple syrup
- 1 cup red apple
- 1 ½ tsp cinnamon
- 1/8 tsp salt
- 2 tbs coconut oil
- 1 egg
- 1 ½ tsp baking powder

DIRECTIONS

1. Mix the dry ingredients in a bowl.
2. In another bowl, whisk the wet ingredients.

3. Add the wet ingredients to the dry ingredients and stir until combined.
4. Refrigerate for 30 minutes.
5. Preheat the oven to 325F.
6. For 15 balls from the dough and place on a lined baking sheet.
7. Bake for 15 minutes.
8. Allow to cool, then serve.

MINT CREAM

Serves: 2

Prep Time: 5 Minutes

Cook Time: 0 Minutes

Total Time: 5 Minutes

INGREDIENTS

- ½ cup coconut cream
- 1/8 tsp peppermint extract
- 3 tbs chocolate chips

- 2 bananas
- Salt

DIRECTIONS

1. Blend all of the ingredients together except for the chocolate chips.
2. Stir in the chocolate chips.
3. Serve immediately.

BLACK BEAN BROWNIES

Serves: **10**

Prep Time: **5** Minutes

Cook Time: **15** Minutes

Total Time: **20** Minutes

INGREDIENTS

- ½ cup maple syrup
- ¼ cup coconut oil

- ½ cup oats
- 2 tsp vanilla extract
- ½ tsp baking powder
- 1 15-ounces can black beans
- ½ cup chocolate chips
- 2 tbs cocoa powder
- ¼ tsp salt

DIRECTIONS

1. Preheat the oven to 350F.
2. Blend all of the ingredients except for the chips until smooth.
3. Stir in the chocolate chips and pour into a pan.
4. Bake for 20 minutes.
5. Allow to cool, cut, then serve.

TURMERIC TEA

Serves: **4**

Prep Time: **5** Minutes

Cook Time: **5** Minutes

Total Time: **10** Minutes

INGREDIENTS

- Black pepper
- ¼ tsp ginger
- ½ tsp cinnamon
- 2 cups milk
- 1 tsp turmeric
- 1 tsp honey

DIRECTIONS

1. Blend all of the ingredients together until smooth.
2. Pour into a saucepan and heat for a few minutes until hot.
3. Serve immediately.

PUMPKIN SPICE LATTE

Serves: **1**

Prep Time: **5** Minutes

Cook Time: **5** Minutes

Total Time: **10** Minutes

INGREDIENTS

- ½ cup almond milk
- Cinnamon
- 1 tsp pumpkin pie spice
- ½ tsp vanilla
- 3 tbs pumpkin puree
- 3 drops stevia
- 8 ounces coffee

DIRECTIONS

1. Heat the almond milk and pumpkin puree until hot.
2. Remove from heat and stir in the vanilla, spices and stevia.
3. Blend the mixture until foamy.

4. Pour coffee into a mug and add the mixture over.
5. Serve sprinkled with cinnamon.

GRANOLA

Serves: **4**
Prep Time: **5** Minutes
Cook Time: **50** Minutes
Total Time: **55** Minutes

INGREDIENTS

- 4 cups rolled oats
- ½ cup chopped hazelnuts
- 2 tbs flax seeds
- 1 cup coconut
- 1/3 cup honey
- ½ cup chopped almonds
- ¼ tsp nutmeg
- ½ tsp salt
- 1/3 cup applesauce

- 1/3 cup apple juice
- 1 cup cranberries
- 3 tbs brown sugar
- ½ tsp cinnamon

DIRECTIONS

1. Preheat the oven to 300F.
2. Mix the oats, flaxseeds, coconut, cinnamon, salt, nutmeg, and brown sugar in a bowl.
3. In another bowl, whisk the applesauce, honey, and apple juice.
4. Pour the liquid mixture over the oats and stir until well coated.
5. Place on a lined baking sheet and cook for 50 minutes, stirring every 10 minutes.
6. Allow to cool, then add the cranberries and serve.

CHOCOLATE MOUSSE

Serves: **4**

Prep Time: **3h 10** Minutes

Cook Time: **5** Minutes

Total Time: **3h 15** Minutes

INGREDIENTS

- 1/3 cup almond milk
- ½ cup cocoa powder
- 1 tbs vanilla
- ¼ tsp salt
- ½ cup chocolate chips
- 4 avocados
- Raspberries
- ½ cup agave

DIRECTIONS

1. Melt the chocolate chips, then set aside.
2. Blend all of the ingredients, including the melted chocolate, until smooth.

3. Spoon into glasses and refrigerate for at least 3 hours.
4. Serve garnished with raspberries.

ICED COFFEE

Serves: 24

Prep Time: 8 Hours

Cook Time: 0 Minutes

Total Time: 8 Hours

INGREDIENTS

- 1 lb coffee
- Milk
- Sweetener
- 8 quarts cold water
- Ice

DIRECTIONS

1. Mix the ground coffee with the water and allow to sit for at least 6 hours.
2. Pour the coffee mixture through a strainer.
3. Allow the coffee liquid to chill in the fridge.
4. Serve with ice, milk and natural sweetener.

KALE ICE POPS

Serves: 4

Prep Time: 5 Hours

Cook Time: 0 Minutes

Total Time: 5 Hours

INGREDIENTS

- 2 cups fruit mix of strawberries, cherries, kale and blueberries
- ¼ cup fruit juice

DIRECTIONS

1. Blend the fruits until smooth.

2. Slowly incorporate the juice.
3. Pour the mixture into ice pop molds.
4. Place in the freezer for at least 5 hours.

MACAROON BARS

Serves: **12**

Prep Time: **5** Minutes

Cook Time: **5** Minutes

Total Time: **10** Minutes

INGREDIENTS

- 1 cup almonds
- ½ tsp cinnamon
- ½ tsp cocoa powder
- Salt
- ¼ cup almond butter
- 2 tbs water
- 1 tsp vanilla
- 1 cup Medjool dates

DIRECTIONS

1. Mix all of the ingredients.
2. Pulse until smooth.
3. Press the dough onto a jellyroll pan.
4. Slice into bars and serve.

CHOCOLATE ICE CREAM

Serves: **4**

Prep Time: **10** Minutes

Cook Time: **0** Minutes

Total Time: **10** Minutes

INGREDIENTS

- 1 tsp vanilla
- ¼ cup cocoa powder
- 1 14-ounces can coconut milk
- ¼ cup honey

DIRECTIONS

1. Blend all of the ingredients in a blender until smooth.
2. Freeze for at least 5 hours.
3. Serve cold.

FATTY LIVER DIET

50+ Side Dishes, Salad and Pasta recipes designed for Fatty Liver Diet

SALAD RECIPES

CHICKEN LIVER SALAD

Serves: **4**

Prep Time: **5** Minutes

Cook Time: **5** Minutes

Total Time: **10** Minutes

INGREDIENTS

- 6 thin slices whole meal bread
- 1 orange
- 1 tablespoon olive oil
- 1 lb. chicken liver
- ¼ cup parsley
- ¼ lb. mixed salad leaves

DIRECTIONS

1. In a bowl mix all ingredients and mix well
2. Serve with dressing

SPICED CHICKEN LIVER SALAD

Serves: **4**

Prep Time: **5** Minutes

Cook Time: **5** Minutes

Total Time: **10** Minutes

INGREDIENTS

- ¾ head iceberg lettuce
- 1 oz. coriander
- 1 pinch salt
- 2 cloves garlic
- 1 onion
- ¼ tsp curry powder
- 1 lb. chicken livers
- 1 tablespoon olive oil

DIRECTIONS

1. **In a bowl add all ingredients and mix well**
2. **Serve with dressing**

CHICKEN LIVER AND BACON SALAD

Serves: 2

Prep Time: 5 Minutes

Cook Time: 5 Minutes

Total Time: 10 Minutes

INGREDIENTS

- 1 onion
- 1 tsp olive oil
- ¼ lb. smoked bacon
- 3 oz. sourdough bread
- 1/3 lb. chicken livers
- 50 ml white wine
- 2 handfuls rocket
- ¼ bunch parsley

DIRECTIONS

1. **In a bowl add all ingredients and mix well**
2. **Serve with dressing**

CHICKEN LIVER SALAD WITH DRESSING

Serves: **2**

Prep Time: **5** Minutes

Cook Time: **5** Minutes

Total Time: **10** Minutes

INGREDIENTS

- 1 oz. chicken livers
- 1 tsp salt
- 1 slice bread
- 2 tablespoons butter
- 5 rashers bacon
- 3 handfuls of salad leaves

DRESSING

- 1 tablespoon cider vinegar
- 1 tsp mustard
- 1 pinch of salt
- 1 tablespoon live oil
- 1 tablespoon walnut oil

DIRECTIONS

1. In a bowl add all ingredients and mix well
2. Serve with dressing

BUTTER & CAULI-COUSCOUS SALAD

Serves: **4**

Prep Time: **5** Minutes

Cook Time: **5** Minutes

Total Time: **10** Minutes

INGREDIENTS

- 2 red beets
- 1 tablespoon lemon juice
- 1 cup cauliflower florets
- ½ cup vegetable stock
- ½ cup orange juice
- 1 tablespoon unsalted butter
- ¼ cup couscous

- 1 tsp orange zest
- 1 tsp salt

DIRECTIONS

1. In a bowl add all ingredients and mix well
2. Serve with dressing

LENTIL AND BRUSSELS SPROUT SALAD

Serves: 4

Prep Time: 5 Minutes

Cook Time: 5 Minutes

Total Time: 10 Minutes

INGREDIENTS

- 2 cups vegetable broth
- 2 bay leaves
- ½ cup apple juice
- 1 cup pecans

- 50 ml maple syrup
- 10 Brussels sprouts
- 2 green onions
- 1 pinch salt

DRESSING
- 4 tablespoons olive oil
- 2 tablespoons apple cider vinegar
- 2 tablespoons yeast
- 2 tablespoons maple syrup

DIRECTIONS

1. **In a bowl add all ingredients and mix well**
2. **Serve with dressing**

CHICKEN CAESAR SALAD

Serves: 2

Prep Time: 5 Minutes

Cook Time: 5 Minutes

Total Time: 10 Minutes

INGREDIENTS

- 2 boneless chicken breast
- 2 tsp olive oil
- ½ tsp salt
- ½ tsp paprika
- ½ tsp pepper
- ¼ tsp dried basil
- ¼ tsp dried oregano
- 3 cups romaine torn
- 1 tomato
- ½ cup salad dressing

DIRECTIONS

1. In a bowl add all ingredients and mix well
2. Serve with dressing

CITRUS SESAME SEED SALAD

Serves: **4**

Prep Time: **5** Minutes

Cook Time: **5** Minutes

Total Time: **10** Minutes

INGREDIENTS

- 1 orange
- 1 lemon
- 1 lime
- 1 pink grapefruit
- 1/3 baby arugula
- ½ lb. feta
- 2 onions
- 1 tablespoon sesame seeds

DRESSING

- juice of 1 lime
- juice of 1 orange
- 1 tablespoon honey
- 1 tablespoon white vinegar
- 1/3 cup olive oil

DIRECTIONS

1. In a bowl add all ingredients and mix well
2. Serve with dressing

PROSCIUTTO SALAD WITH ORANGE VINAIRETTE

Serves: **4**

Prep Time: **5** Minutes

Cook Time: **5** Minutes

Total Time: **10** Minutes

INGREDIENTS

- 1 oakleaf lettuce
- 3 ripe figs
- ¼ lb. prosciutto
- 12 basil leaves
- 2 oz. parmesan

ORANGE VINAIGRETTE
- 1 tablespoon orange juice
- 1 tsp balsamic vinegar
- 1 tsp mustard
- ¼ tsp orange zest
- ½ cup olive oil

DIRECTIONS

1. In a bowl add all ingredients and mix well
2. Serve with dressing

COLESLAW

Serves: **4**

Prep Time: **5** Minutes

Cook Time: **5** Minutes

Total Time: **10** Minutes

INGREDIENTS

- 1 carrot
- ½ red cabbage
- 1 handful parsley
- 2 scallions
- 2 tablespoon mayonnaise
- salt

DIRECTIONS

1. **In a bowl add all ingredients and mix well**
2. **Serve with dressing**

BLUE CHEESE AND FIG SALAD

Serves: **4**

Prep Time: **5** Minutes

Cook Time: **5** Minutes

Total Time: **10** Minutes

INGREDIENTS

- ½ cup pine nuts
- ¼ apple
- ¾ cup blue cheese
- 6 oz. salad greens

DRESSING

- 1 tsp Dijon mustard
- 2 tablespoons balsamic vinegar
- ¼ cup olive oil
- 1 heaping tablespoon fig jam
- 1 garlic clove

DIRECTIONS

1. In a bowl add all ingredients and mix well
2. Serve with dressing

VEGAN WHITE BEAN SALAD

Serves: **4**

Prep Time: **5** Minutes

Cook Time: **5** Minutes

Total Time: **10** Minutes

INGREDIENTS

- 2 cans white beans
- 2 cloves garlic
- 1 onion
- ¼ cup parsley
- 2 tablespoons olive oil
- 2 tomatoes
- ½ cup black olives
- 2 tablespoons wine vinegar
- lemon juice for 1 lemon
- 1 pinch of salt

DIRECTIONS

1. **In a bowl add all ingredients and mix well**
2. **Serve with dressing**

JAPANESE VEGA SALAD DRESSING

Serves: **4**

Prep Time: **5** Minutes

Cook Time: **5** Minutes

Total Time: **10** Minutes

INGREDIENTS

- ½ cup miso
- 1 tablespoon rice vinegar
- 1 tablespoon soy sauce
- 1 tablespoon sesame oil
- ¼ tsp ginger
- 1 tablespoon water

DIRECTIONS

1. **In a bowl add all ingredients and mix well**
2. **Serve with dressing**

ROASTED CAULIFLOWER SALAD

Serves: **4**

Prep Time: **5** Minutes

Cook Time: **5** Minutes

Total Time: **10** Minutes

INGREDIENTS

- 1 head roasted cauliflower
- 1 tablespoon canola
- 1 tsp turmeric
- 1 tsp cumin
- 1 pinch of salt
- ½ red onion
- 1 tablespoon lemon juice
- 1 tsp honey
- ½ cup pomegranate seeds
- 2 heaping tablespoons parsley

DIRECTIONS

1. In a bowl add all ingredients and mix well
2. Serve with dressing

BROCCOLI SALAD WITH BACON

Serves: **4**

Prep Time: **5** Minutes

Cook Time: **5** Minutes

Total Time: **10** Minutes

INGREDIENTS

- 10 bacon
- 2 broccoli crowns
- 1 red onion
- ¼ cup raisins

DRESSING

- 1 cup mayonnaise
- 1 tablespoon balsamic vinegar
- 1 tsp sugar

DIRECTIONS

1. In a bowl add all ingredients and mix well
2. Serve with dressing

RED POTATO SALAD

Serves: **4**

Prep Time: **5** Minutes

Cook Time: **5** Minutes

Total Time: **10** Minutes

INGREDIENTS

- 1 lb. red potatoes
- 3 eggs
- 2 ribs celery
- ¼ cup red onion
- 3 green onions
- 2 tablespoons diced dill pickle
- ½ cup sour cream
- 1/3 cup mayonnaise
- 1 tablespoon tarragon vinegar
- 1 tsp mustard
- ¼ tsp salt
- ¼ tsp pepper

DIRECTIONS

1. In a bowl add all ingredients and mix well
2. Serve with dressing

TANGY RED CABBAGE SLAW

Serves: **4**

Prep Time: **5** Minutes

Cook Time: **5** Minutes

Total Time: **10** Minutes

INGREDIENTS

- 1 cup mayonnaise
- 2 tablespoons sugar
- 2 tablespoons apple cider vinegar
- 1 head red cabbage
- 1 red onion
- 1/3 cup raisins
- 3 tablespoons pecans

DIRECTIONS

1. In a bowl add all ingredients and mix well
2. Serve with dressing

PIZZA RECIPES

GRAIN-FREE PIZZA CRUST

Serves: **4**

Prep Time: **15** Minutes

Cook Time: **15** Minutes

Total Time: **30** Minutes

INGREDIENTS

- 2 eggs
- 2 tablespoons apple sauce
- ¼ cup coconut flour
- ½ cup almond flour
- ½ tsp salt
- ½ tsp dried basil

DIRECTIONS

1. In a food processor add the eggs and process until smooth
2. Add salt, coconut flour, applesauce, almond flour and mix well
3. Mix until it forms a ball in the processor

4. Scrap the dough together into a ball, put the dough onto the parchment paper
5. Bake at 350 F for 15 minutes
6. Remove from oven and serve the pizza crust

PIZZA WITH SPICY CHICKEN LIVER

Serves: **4**

Prep Time: **10** Minutes

Cook Time: **20** Minutes

Total Time: **30** Minutes

INGREDIENTS

- ½ cup water
- 1 envelope active dry yeast
- 1 cup water
- 1 tablespoon olive oil
- 3 cups bread flour
- 1 tsp salt
- 1 tsp vegetable oil

DIRECTIONS

1. Sprinkle water in yeast and let it stand for a couple of minutes
2. Add oil and stir to combine
3. In a blender add flour and salt and blend for 30-45 seconds
4. Pour liquid ingredients and continue to blend until it the dough is formed
5. Put dough into an oiled bowl, cover and let it stand for 1-2 hours
6. Over dough add toppings like, red pepper flakes, onion, olives, chicken livers and cheddar cheese
7. Preheat the oven at 475 F
8. Bake pizza for 15-18 minutes or until golden brown
9. When ready remove and serve

DETOX CAULIFLOWER PIZZA

Serves: **4**

Prep Time: **10** Minutes

Cook Time: **20** Minutes

Total Time: **30** Minutes

INGREDIENTS

- ½ head cauliflower
- 1 tablespoon almond meal
- 1 tsp oregano
- 1 egg

SAUCE

- 1 tomato
- 1 head garlic
- 1 handful basil
- 1 drizzle olive oil

DIRECTIONS

1. Preheat the oven at 325 F

2. In a blender add chopped cauliflower and blend for 60 seconds, place it in a bowl and microwave for 4-5 minutes
3. Add the rest of the ingredients to the bowl and mix well
4. Spread mixture on a cookie sheet lined with parchment paper and bake for 12-15 minutes
5. In a blender add all ingredients for the sauce and blend until smooth
6. Add to your pan on the stove and cook
7. Add toppings like red pepper, mushrooms, zucchini, spinach
8. Bake for another 8-10 minutes
9. When ready remove and serve

CAULIFLOWER CRUST PIZAA

Serves: 4

Prep Time: 10 Minutes

Cook Time: 20 Minutes

Total Time: 30 Minutes

INGREDIENTS

- 1 lb. ground beef
- 1 egg
- 1 tsp parsley
- 1 tsp dried basil
- ¼ tsp salt
- ½ tsp pepper
- ¼ cup tomato puree
- 1 tsp tomato paste
- ¼ red pepper
- 1 tsp dried basil
- ¼ cup olives
- 5 slices prosciutto
- 4 oz. parmesan
- 1 handful fresh basil

DIRECTIONS

1. Preheat the oven to 430 F
2. In a bowl add salt, mince, egg, basil, pepper, parsley and mix well
3. Roll into a ball and place on a baking tray
4. Bake for 12-15 minutes
5. Mix the tomato paste with tomato puree and spread across the base
6. Top with peppers, prosciutto, parmesan, olives and bake for another 8-10 minutes

7. Remove from the oven, top with basil leaves and serve

LIVER DETOXIYING PIZZA

Serves: **4**

Prep Time: **10** Minutes

Cook Time: **20** Minutes

Total Time: **30** Minutes

INGREDIENTS

- 1 gluten-free pizza crust

SAUCE

- 1 tablespoons tomato paste
- 1 tablespoon balsamic vinegar
- 1 tsp honey
- 1 clove garlic

TOPPINGS

- 1 tsp olive oil
- ¼ onion
- 1 cup shiitake mushrooms
- ¼ bell pepper
- ½ cup jarred artichokes
- 1 tablespoon sun-dried tomatoes
- 1 tablespoon balsamic vinegar

DIRECTIONS

1. Preheat the oven to 350 F
2. Cook your pizza crust fro 12-15 minutes
3. In a pan add olive oil, mushrooms and the rest of the toppings and cook for 5-7 minutes on low heat
4. In a bowl prepare add all the ingredients for the sauce and mix well
5. Remove pizza crust from the oven, add pizza sauce and toppings
6. Place pizza back in the oven and bake for 8-10 minutes
7. When ready, remove and serve

CAULIFLOWER PIZZA CRUST

Serves: **4**

Prep Time: **10** Minutes

Cook Time: **30** Minutes

Total Time: **40** Minutes

INGREDIENTS

- 1 cauliflower head
- 1 cup parmesan
- ¼ tsp Italian seasoning
- 1 clove garlic
- ¼ tsp salt
- 1 egg
- olive oil
- 1 cup mozzarella
- ¼ cup marinara sauce
- ½ cup basil leaves
- 1 tomato

DIRECTIONS

1. **Preheat the oven to 450 F**

2. In a blender add cauliflower and blend until finely ground
3. In a bowl add parmesan, cauliflower, garlic, egg, Italian seasoning, salt and mix well
4. Spread the cauliflower mixture on a parchment paper and bake until the crust is barely golden, 12-15 minutes
5. Remove from the oven, sprinkle with mozzarella, marinara sauce, tomato slices and bake for another 6-8 minutes
6. When ready, remove and serve

EGGPLANT HUMMUS PIZZA

Serves: 2

Prep Time: **10** Minutes

Cook Time: **30** Minutes

Total Time: **40** Minutes

INGREDIENTS

- 1 cup gluten-free flour
- 1 tsp psllium husk powder

- ½ tsp salt
- ¼ tsp active dry yeast
- ¼ tsp olive oil
- ¾ cup water
- 2 cups lentil hummus
- 7 slices eggplant
- 4 sweet peppers sliced
- 6 olives sliced

DIRECTIONS

1. Preheat the oven at 350 F
2. In a bowl whisk psyllium husk, yeast, salt, flour and mix well
3. Add olive oil, water, mix and let the dough rise for 2-3 hours
4. Transfer the dough onto a surface and roll the dough to form a smooth ball and then flatten the ball to form a disk
5. Fold the pizza dough disk in half, and then again, form a triangle
6. Transfer onto a dusted pizza pan
7. Bake for 15-18 minutes or until barely golden
8. Remove from the oven, spoon the lentil hummus in the center, eggplant slices, olives, peppers and sprinkle with cheese on top
9. Bake for another 6-8 minutes
10. When ready remove and serve

RAW SQUASH HUMMUS PIZZA

Serves: **4**

Prep Time: **10** Minutes

Cook Time: **35** Minutes

Total Time: **45** Minutes

INGREDIENTS

CRUST

- 1/2 butternut squash
- 1 garlic clove
- 1 tablespoon ground flaxseed
- ¾ cup flaxseed
- 1 tsp salt
- 1 tsp thyme

SQUASH HUMMUS

- 2 cups butternut squash
- 1 cup raw walnuts
- 1 tsp thyme
- 1 garlic clove
- 2 tsp cumin
- water as needed
- spinach leaves

- 6 tomato slices

DIRECTIONS

1. Preheat the oven to 375 F
2. In a blender add all ingredients for the crust and blend until smooth
3. Add water if necessary and blend again
4. Spread batter into a circle on a lined dehydrator tray and dehydrate for 16-18 hours
5. For squash mush combine all ingredients and blend until smooth
6. Spread the hummus over the crust and top with tomatoes, onion, spinach leaves
7. When ready, serve!

ZUCCHINI PIZZA CRUST

Serves: *4*
Prep Time: *10* Minutes
Cook Time: *30* Minutes
Total Time: *40* Minutes

INGREDIENTS

- 4 zucchini
- 2 tsp salt
- 2 cups almond flour
- 2 tablespoons coconut flour
- 3 eggs
- 2 ½ cups parmesan cheese
- 1 tsp red pepper flakes
- 1 tsp dried oregano

DIRECTIONS

1. Shred the zucchini, sprinkle with salt and set aside
2. Preheat the oven to 400 F
3. Mix zucchini with remaining ingredients
4. Place the dough over a baking sheet and spread evenly
5. Pop the pizza crust in the oven for 30 minutes or until golden brown
6. When ready, remove and serve

SPINACH PESTO PIZZA

Serves: **4**

Prep Time: **10** Minutes

Cook Time: **20** Minutes

Total Time: **30** Minutes

INGREDIENTS

CRUST
- **½ cup hemp seeds**
- **1 cup walnuts**
- **1 tsp salt**
- **1 tsp basil**
- **1 tablespoon maple syrup**
- **1 tablespoon water**
- **¼ onion**

PESTO
- **4 cups spinach**
- **¼ cup pine nuts**
- **1 garlic clove**
- **¼ tsp salt**
- **¼ cup water**

TOPPINGS
- **3-4 mushrooms**

- 1 bell pepper
- 1 tomato
- 1 tsp tamari

DIRECTIONS

1. In a blender add all ingredients for the crust and blend until smooth
2. Spread batter into a circle on a lined dehydrator tray and dehydrate for 4-5 hours
3. In a blender add all ingredients for pesto and blend until it reaches pesto consistency
4. Spread pesto over pizza crust and add toppings
5. When ready, serve

RAW VEGAN PIZZA

Serves: *4*
Prep Time: *10* Minutes
Cook Time: *30* Minutes
Total Time: *40* Minutes

INGREDIENTS

- cashew cheese as needed
- tomato sauce as needed

CRUST

- 6 tomatoes
- 1 zucchini pulp
- 1 red bell pepper
- 1 onion
- 1 tablespoon flax seeds
- 2 tablespoon sesame seeds
- 1 tablespoon ground sunflower seeds
- 1 tablespoon tamari sauce
- 1 tablespoon olive oil

TOPPINGS

- arugula
- 4-5 cherry tomatoes
- 3-4 mushrooms
- 4-5 black olives

DIRECTIONS

1. In a blender add all ingredients for the crust and blend until smooth
2. Spread batter into a circle on a lined dehydrator tray and dehydrate for 10-12 hours
3. Cut the ingredients for toppings in thin slices
4. Place tomato sauce, cashew cheese and toppings over pizza crust

SIDE DISHES

SESAME PORK TACOS

Serves: **4**

Prep Time: **5** Minutes

Cook Time: **15** Minutes

Total Time: **25** Minutes

INGREDIENTS

- 1 cup cucumber slices
- 5 radishes
- ½ cup red wine vinegar
- 3 tsp sugar
- 1 tablespoon olive oil
- 3 scallions
- 1 cup red cabbage
- 1 lb. ground pork
- 2 tsp garlic powder
- 2 tablespoons sesame oil
- 2 tablespoons soy sauce
- 1 tsp Sriracha
- 10 tortillas
- 1 tsp cilantro

- ¼ cup sour cream
- 1 pinch of salt

DIRECTIONS

1. In a bowl add radishes, cucumbers, vinegar, 1 tsp sugar and salt, stir well to combine
2. In a pan add oil, scallions, cabbage and cook for 4-5 minutes
3. Add pork, sugar, garlic powder and cook for another 4-5 minutes
4. Add soy sauce, sesame oil and stir to combine
5. Spread sour cream in the center of your tortilla, add pork filling and sprinkle cilantro, radishes and top with meat mixture

WATERMELON GAZPACHO

Serves: 3
Prep Time: **10** Minutes
Cook Time: **10** Minutes
Total Time: **20** Minutes

INGREDIENTS

- 2 cups ripe watermelon
- 1 red pepper
- ¼ onion
- 3 tablespoons red wine vinegar
- 6 tablespoons cranberry juice
- Italian basil leaves as needed

DIRECTIONS

1. Puree all ingredients, except the basil, until smooth
2. Refrigerate to chill
3. Serve garnished with basil, onion, tomato or cucumber

VEGETARIAN MINESTRONE SOUP

Serves: 5
Prep Time: *10* Minutes

Cook Time: *40* Minutes

Total Time: *50* Minutes

INGREDIENTS

- 1 tablespoon olive oil
- ¾ cup onion
- 2 ½ cups water
- 2 cups zucchini
- 1 cup sliced carrots
- 1 cup beans
- ¼ cup celery
- 2 tablespoons basil
- 1/3 tsp oregano
- ¼ tsp salt
- ¼ tsp black pepper
- 1 can plum tomatoes
- 2 cloves garlic
- ½ cup uncooked pasta

DIRECTIONS

1. In a saucepan add oil, onion and sauté for 4-5 minutes
2. Add remaining ingredients and bring to a boil
3. Reduce heat and simmer on low heat for 20-25 minutes
4. Add pasta and cook until pasta is al dente for 10-12 minutes
5. When ready, remove from heat and serve

LIME GRILLED CORN

Serves: 3

Prep Time: 5 Minutes

Cook Time: 15 Minutes

Total Time: 20 Minutes

INGREDIENTS

- 3 ears of corn
- 2 tablespoons mayonnaise
- 2 tablespoons squeezed lime juice
- ½ tsp chili powder
- 1 pinch of salt

DIRECTIONS

1. Place corn onto the grill and cook for 5-6 minutes or until the kernels being to brown
2. Turn every few minutes until all sides are slightly charred
3. In a bowl mix the rest of ingredients
4. Spread a light coating of the mixture onto each cob and serve

MACADAMIA DIP WITH VEGETABLES

Serves: **4**

Prep Time: **10** Minutes

Cook Time: **30** Minutes

Total Time: **40** Minutes

INGREDIENTS

- 6 oz. squash
- ½ bunch basil
- ¼ cup macadamia nuts
- 1 tablespoon olive oil
- ¼ lemon
- ¼ tsp ground smoked paprika
- salt
- vegetable sticks

DIRECTIONS

1. Preheat the oven to 350 F
2. Cut the squash into chunks and roast for 25-30 minutes
3. In a food processor add the basil leaves, lemon zest, macadamia nuts, squash pieces and salt

4. Serve with vegetable sticks: cucumber, carrots, tomatoes and green pepper

GINGERSNAPS

Serves: **6**

Prep Time: **10** Minutes

Cook Time: **15** Minutes

Total Time: **25** Minutes

INGREDIENTS

- 1 cup white whole wheat flour
- 1 cornstarch
- 1 tsp baking powder
- 1 tsp ground ginger
- ½ tsp ground cinnamon
- ¼ tsp nutmeg
- ¼ tsp ground cloves
- ½ tsp salt
- 1 tablespoon unsalted butter

- 1 egg white
- 2 tsp vanilla stevia
- ½ cup nonfat milk
- ½ cup molasses
- 1 tsp vanilla extract

DIRECTIONS

1. Preheat the oven to 350 F
2. In a bowl whisk together the cornstarch, ginger, baking powder, cinnamon, nutmeg, cloves and salt and flour
3. In another bowl mix vanilla extract, egg, butter, stevia, molasses and milk
4. Add in the flour mixture and stir until fully incorporated
5. Divide dough into 14-16 portions and roll each into a ball
6. Place onto a baking sheet and press it down into the cookie dough
7. Bake for 8-10 minutes
8. When ready, remove and serve

TURKEY & VEGGIES STUFFED PEPPERS

Serves: *4*

Prep Time: *10* Minutes

Cook Time: *40* Minutes

Total Time: *50* Minutes

INGREDIENTS

- 4 red bell peppers
- 1 lb. ground turkey
- 1 tablespoon olive oil
- ¼ onion
- 1 cup mushrooms 1 zucchini
- ½ green bell pepper
- ½ yellow bell pepper
- 1 cup spinach
- 1 can diced tomatoes
- 1 tsp Italian seasoning
- ¼ tsp garlic powder
- 1 pinch of salt

DIRECTIONS

1. **Preheat the oven to 325 F**

2. In a pot bring water to boil, add pepper and cook for 5-6 minutes
3. In a skillet cook the turkey until brown and set aside
4. In another pan add onion, olive oil, mushrooms, zucchini, green, yellow pepper, spinach and cook until tender
5. Add remaining ingredients to the turkey and cook until done
6. Stuff the peppers with the mixture and place them into a casserole dish
7. Bake for 15-18 minutes or until done

QUINOA TACO MEAT

Serves: 6
Prep Time: *10* Minutes
Cook Time: *50* Minutes
Total Time: *60* Minutes

INGREDIENTS

- 1 cup red quinoa

- 1 cup vegetable broth
- ¾ cup water

SEASONING

- ¼ cup salsa
- 1 tablespoon yeast
- 1 tsp cumin
- 1 tsp chili powder
- ¼ tsp garlic powder
- ½ tsp black pepper
- ½ tsp salt
- 1 tablespoon olive oil
-

DIRECTIONS

1. In a saucepan add quinoa and cook for 5-6 minutes
2. Add water, vegetable broth and bring to a boil
3. Reduce heat to low and cook for 20-22 minutes or until liquid is absorbed
4. Add quinoa to a mixing bowl, remaining ingredients and toss to combine
5. Bake for 25-30 minutes or until golden brown
6. When ready remove and serve with taco salads, enchiladas or nachos

KALE CHIPS

Serves: 6

Prep Time: 10 Minutes

Cook Time: 25 Minutes

Total Time: 35 Minutes

INGREDIENTS

- 1 bunch of kale
- 1 tablespoon olive oil
- 1 tsp salt

DIRECTIONS

1. Preheat the oven to 325 F
2. Chop the kale into chip size pieces
3. Put pieces into a bowl tops with olive oil and salt
4. Spread the leaves in a single layer onto a parchment paper
5. Bake for 20-25 minutes
6. When ready, remove and serve

CHICKEN AND BROWN RICE PASTA

Serves: **2**

Prep Time: **10** Minutes

Cook Time: **15** Minutes

Total Time: **25** Minutes

INGREDIENTS

- 1 cup cooked rice pasta
- 1 chicken breast
- ¼ cup no sugar marinara sauce
- ½ cup tomatoes
- parsley for serving
- 1 tsp olive oil

DIRECTIONS

1. In a skillet cook the pasta according to the package directions
2. Drain and rinse the pasta
3. Add cooked chicken breast, marinara sauce and serve

PHILLY CHEESE STEAK

Serves: **4**

Prep Time: **5** Minutes

Cook Time: **20** Minutes

Total Time: **25** Minutes

INGREDIENTS

- 2 tsp olive oil
- 1 onion
- 3 portobello mushrooms
- 1 red bell pepper
- 1 tsp dried oregano
- ¼ tsp ground pepper
- 1 tablespoon all-purpose flour
- ½ cup vegetable broth
- 1 tablespoon soy sauce
- 2 oz. vegan cheese
- 3 whole-wheat rolls

DIRECTIONS

1. In a skillet add onion, pepper, bell pepper, oregano and cook until soft

2. Reduce heat, sprinkle flour, soy sauce, broth and bring to a simmer
3. Remove from heat, add cheese slices on top and let it stand until fully melted
4. Divide into 3-4 portions and serve

CAULIFLOWER WINGS

Serves: **4**

Prep Time: **10** Minutes

Cook Time: **50** Minutes

Total Time: **60** Minutes

INGREDIENTS

- 1 head cauliflower
- ¼ unsweetened almond milk
- ¼ cup water
- ¾ rice flour
- 1 tsp garlic powder
- 1 tsp onion powder

- 1 tsp cumin
- 1 tsp paprika
- ½ tsp salt
- ¼ tsp ground pepper
- bbq sauce

VINEGAR SAUCE
- 1 tablespoon vegan butter
- 2 tablespoons apple cider vinegar
- 1 tablespoon water
- 1 pinch of salt

DIRECTIONS

1. Preheat the oven to 425 F
2. Mix all wing ingredients in a bowl and submerge each cauliflower floret into the mix
3. Place florets on a prepare baking sheet
4. Bake for 10 minutes, flip and bake for another 10 minutes or until golden brown
5. Remove the cauliflower from the oven and serve with vinegar sauce
6. When ready season with pepper and salt and serve

ROASTED BOK CHOY

Serves: **4**

Prep Time: **5** Minutes

Cook Time: **15** Minutes

Total Time: **20** Minutes

INGREDIENTS

- 5 heads baby bok choy
- olive oil
- 1 tsp pepper
- 1 tsp salt

DIRECTIONS

1. Preheat the oven to 425 F
2. Cut each bok choy in half lengthwise and place on a baking sheet
3. Drizzle with olive oil, pepper and salt
4. Bake for 10-12 minutes, flip and bake for another 8-10 minutes
5. When ready remove and serve

ROASTED TURKEY

Serves: **12**

Prep Time: **10** Minutes

Cook Time: **120** Minutes

Total Time: **130** Minutes

INGREDIENTS

- 12 lbs. turkey
- 4 tablespoons melted
- 1 tsp pepper
- salt as needed

DIRECTIONS

1. Preheat the oven at 400 F
2. Prepare the turkey to be roasted
3. Brush the breast and legs of the turkey with butter, salt, pepper and arrange it breast-side down on a rack
4. Roast for 60-75 minutes
5. Remove from the oven, tip the juice from the cavity of the turkey into the pan
6. Flip the turkey breast-side up and place back in the oven at 375 F for another 60 minutes

MAPLE-ROASTED SWEET POTATOES

Serves: *12*

Prep Time: *10* Minutes

Cook Time: *50* Minutes

Total Time: *60* Minutes

INGREDIENTS

- ½ cup maple syrup
- 1 tablespoon butter
- 1 tablespoon lemon juice
- ¼ tsp salt
- 2 lbs. sweet potatoes
- 1 red onion

DIRECTIONS

1. Preheat the oven to 425 F
2. In a bowl combine butter, lemon juice, maple syrup, salt and pepper
3. Place sweet potatoes and onions into a baking dish
4. Pour maple syrup mixture over the potatoes and bake for 12-15 minutes or until golden brown
5. When ready, remove and and serve

CAULIFLOWER FRITTERS

Serves: **8**

Prep Time: **10** Minutes

Cook Time: **30** Minutes

Total Time: **40** Minutes

INGREDIENTS

- 1 head of cauliflower
- ¼ tsp chili powder
- 2 cloves garlic
- 2 tablespoons cilantro
- 1 tsp salt
- ¼ tsp black pepper
- 2 eggs
- 3 tablespoons cornmeal
- ½ cup flour
- 4 tablespoons nutritional yeast

DIRECTIONS

1. Cook cauliflower florets by steaming for 5-6 minutes
2. Mix the cauliflower with chili powder, cilantro, garlic, pepper and salt

3. In another bowl beat the egg, add cauliflower mixture, flour, corn meal and yeast
4. Add ¼ cup of the mixture to the pan and press down the fritter
5. Cook until golden brown for 3-4 minutes per side
6. When ready, remove and serve

PEACH CRUMBLE

Serves: *8*
Prep Time: *10* Minutes

Cook Time: *40* Minutes

Total Time: *50* Minutes

INGREDIENTS

- 3 peaches
- 2 tablespoons cornstarch
- 1 tsp almond extract
- 1 tsp cinnamon
- ¾ cup old-fashioned oats

- ½ cup whole wheat flour
- 2 tablespoons agave

DIRECTIONS

1. Preheat the oven to 325 F
2. In a bowl mix cornstarch, almond extract, peaches and ½ cinnamon
3. In another bowl mix flour, oats and remaining cinnamon
4. Add in agave and mix well
5. Spread mixture into a baking dish and sprinkle oat crumbs on top
6. Bake for 35-40 minutes or until mixture turns crunchy
7. When ready remove and serve

GREEK MIXED VEGETABLES

Serves: **6**

Prep Time: **10** Minutes

Cook Time: **90** Minutes

Total Time: **100** Minutes

INGREDIENTS

- ½ cup olive oil
- 1 eggplant
- 1 onion
- 2 garlic cloves
- 1 lb. potatoes
- 5 tomatoes
- 10 cherry tomatoes
- 1 cup tomato passata
- 1 cup water
- 1 tablespoon dried oregano
- 1 tablespoon parsley
- 1 tsp salt

DIRECTIONS

1. Preheat the oven to 400 F
2. In a frying pan add olive oil, eggplant and cook for 6-7 minutes
3. Add garlic, onion and sauté for 5-6 minutes
4. Add potato, zucchini, passata, tomatoes and water
5. Sprinkle with oregano, parley, pepper and salt
6. Mix well and transfer to a baking dish, drizzle with olive oil and bake for 45-55 minutes or until the top has browned
7. When ready remove and serve

CHICKEN BURGER

Serves: *4*

Prep Time: *5* Minutes

Cook Time: *15* Minutes

Total Time: *20* Minutes

INGREDIENTS

- 1 lb. chicken meat
- 2 cups bread crumbs
- ½ cup low-fat milk
- 2 tablespoons grated onion
- ¼ tsp black pepper
- ¼ tsp salt
- 1 tsp olive oil

DIRECTIONS

1. Place chicken in a bowl and fold in bread crumbs, cayenne, onion, salt and pepper
2. Divide chicken meat into 4 piles and shape into patties
3. Coat each patty with bread crumbs
4. Fry the patty for 4-5 per side or until golde

TURKEY MEATLOAF

Serves: *8*

Prep Time: *10* Minutes

Cook Time: *90* Minutes

Total Time: *100* Minutes

INGREDIENTS

- ¼ cup oats
- ½ cup milk
- 1 onion
- 2 lbs. ground turkey breast
- ½ cup red bell pepper
- 2 eggs
- 2 tsp Worcestershire sauce
- ½ cup ketchup
- ¼ tsp salt
- 1 can tomato sauce

DIRECTIONS

1. **Preheat the oven to 375 F**
2. **In a bowl stir in oats milk and let it soak for a couple of minutes**

3. In another bowl combine the ingredients except tomato sauce
4. Transfer the mixture to a baking dish and shape into a loaf
5. Pour tomato sauce over the meatloaf
6. Bake for 60 minutes
7. When ready remove and serve

PASTA & NOODLES

ROASTED CHICKPEAS

Serves: 6
Prep Time: 5 Minutes
Cook Time: 50 Minutes
Total Time: 55 Minutes

INGREDIENTS

- 2 cans chickpeas
- ¼ tsp salt
- 2 tablespoons olive oil

DIRECTIONS

1. Preheat the oven to 400 F
2. Place the chickpeas on a baking sheet and toss with olive oil until they are coated
3. Sprinkle with salt and spread the chickpeas out
4. Bake for 45-55 minutes or until crispy
5. When ready remove and serve

CHICKEN LETTUCE WRAPS

Serves: **4**

Prep Time: **10** Minutes

Cook Time: **15** Minutes

Total Time: **25** Minutes

INGREDIENTS

- 1 tsp salt
- 1 lb. ground chicken
- 2 cloves garlic
- ¼ onion
- ½ cup hoisin sauce
- 1 tablespoon soy sauce
- 1 tablespoon wine vinegar
- 1 tablespoon ginger
- 1 tsp Sriracha
- 1 can chestnuts
- 2 green onion
- 1 carrot
- 1 heat butter lettuce

DIRECTIONS

1. **In a saucepan add olive oil, ground chicken and cook for 4-5 minutes**

2. Stir in onion, garlic, hoisin sauce, wine vinegar, soy sauce, ginger, Sriracha until onions are translucent
3. Stir in water chestnuts and season with salt and pepper
4. When ready spoon chicken mixture into the center of a lettuce leaf and top with carrot

TURMERIC RICE

Serves: 6

Prep Time: 20 Minutes

Cook Time: 60 Minutes

Total Time: 80 Minutes

INGREDIENTS

- 1 tsp coconut oil
- ¼ cup onion
- 1 cup brown rice
- ½ cup golden raisins
- 1 tsp fresh turmeric
- 2 cloves garlic

- 2 cups vegetable broth
- 1 pinch of salt

DIRECTIONS

1. In a saucepan add coconut oil, onions and sauce for 4-5 minutes
2. Add raisins, turmeric, rice and garlic, toss to coat
3. Sauté for 2-3 minutes and slowly bring saucepan to a boil
4. Reduce heat and cook for 40-45 minutes or until rice is tender
5. When ready season with salt, pepper and serve

ROASTED BEET NOODLES WITH PESTO

Serves: 3

Prep Time: 10 Minutes

Cook Time: 15 Minutes

Total Time: 25 Minutes

INGREDIENTS

- 2 beets
- olive oil
- 2 cups baby kale

PESTO

- 2 cups basil leaves
- ½ cup Pinenuts
- ½ cup olive oil
- ¼ tsp salt
- ½ tsp pepper
- 1 clove garlic

DIRECTIONS

1. Preheat the oven to 400 F
2. On a baking sheet spread out the beet noodles and bake for 8-10 minutes
3. In a bowl mix all pesto ingredients and place in a blender, blend until smooth
4. Toss beets with pesto, kale and serve

AVOCADO PESTO NOODLES

Serves: 5

Prep Time: 10 Minutes

Cook Time: 30 Minutes

Total Time: 40 Minutes

INGREDIENTS

- 2 zucchini
- 1 avocado
- 1 handful basil
- juice from ½ lemon
- 1 garlic clove
- 2 tablespoons olive oil
- 1 tablespoon water
- 1 tsp salt

DIRECTIONS

1. Make zucchini noodles and steam noodles until soft
2. In a food processor mix the remaining ingredients and process until smooth
3. When ready, serve noodles with sauce

BUTTERNUT SQUASH PASTA

Serves: **4**

Prep Time: **10** Minutes

Cook Time: **30** Minutes

Total Time: **40** Minutes

INGREDIENTS

- 1 butternut squash
- 1 tablespoon olive oil
- ½ cup bacon
- ½ cup cashews
- 1 clove garlic
- ½ cup almond milk
- ½ tsp salt
- ¼ tsp pepper
- ½ cup peas
- 1 tablespoon parsley

DIRECTIONS

1. Preheat the oven to 375 F
2. Spiralize butternut squash into noodles
3. Place on a baking sheet and toss with olive oil

4. Bake for 8-10 minutes
5. In a bowl mix remaining, except peas, and place in a blender, blend until smooth
6. Pour the sauce into a skillet with peas, add butternut squash pasta and toss to coat
7. Top with parsley and serve

LEMON PASTA WITH SHRIMP

Serves: 5
Prep Time: 10 Minutes
Cook Time: 30 Minutes
Total Time: 40 Minutes

INGREDIENTS

- 1 box gluten-free linguini
- 1 tablespoon garlic-infused olive oil
- 3 tablespoons butter
- 1 lb. shrimp
- 1 tsp Italian seasoning

- ½ tsp red pepper flakes
- 3 cups spinach
- juice of ½ lemon
- 1 tablespoon parsley

DIRECTIONS

1. Cook pasta according to package instructions
2. Drain and toss with olive oil
3. In a pot add shrimp and cook in melted butter
4. Add red pepper flakes, Italian seasoning, spinach and cook until done
5. Add shrimp to pasta mixture, top with lemon juice, herbs, pepper and serve

FATTY LIVER DIET

50+ Smoothies, Dessert and Breakfast recipes designed for Fatty Liver Diet

BREAKFAST

PUMPKIN BAKED OATMEAL

Serves: **6**

Prep Time: **10** Minutes

Cook Time: **30** Minutes

Total Time: **40** Minutes

INGREDIENTS

- ½ cup pumpkin puree
- 2 batches flax eggs
- 1/3 cup maple syrup
- 2 tablespoons coconut oil
- ½ tsp salt
- 1 tsp pumpkin pie spice
- ¼ tsp cinnamon
- 2 cups dairy-free milk
- 2 cups gluten-free rolled oats
- 1/3 cup pecans
- 1/3 cup frozen cranberries
- 2 tablespoons coconut sugar

DIRECTIONS

1. Preheat the oven to 325 F
2. In a bowl prepare flax eggs, add pumpkin puree, salt, maple syrup, oil, pumpkin pie spice, cinnamon and whisk to combine
3. Add milk, pecans, oats and stir to combine
4. Transfer to a baking dish and top with pecans
5. Sprinkle with coconut sugar and cranberries
6. Bake for 30-35 minutes or until golden brown
7. When ready remove and serve

BUCKWHEAT GRANOLA

Serves: *18*
Prep Time: *10* Minutes
Cook Time: *30* Minutes
Total Time: *40* Minutes

INGREDIENTS

- 1 cup buckwheat groats

- 1 cup gluten-free oats
- 1/3 cup raw nuts
- ¼ cup unsweetened coconut flakes
- 2 tablespoons chia seeds
- 2 tablespoons coconut sugar
- ¼ tsp salt
- 1/3 ground cinnamon
- ¼ cup olive oil
- ¼ cup maple syrup
- 2 tablespoons seed butter
- ½ cup dried fruit

DIRECTIONS

1. Preheat the oven to 325 F
2. In a bowl add oats, nuts, buckwheat groats, coconut, coconut sugar, chia seeds, cinnamon and salt
3. In a saucepan add olive oil, maple syrup, nut butter and pour over the dry ingredients and mix well
4. Spread the mixture evenly onto a baking sheet and bake for 25-28 minutes
5. Add dried fruits and store in the refrigerator

FRUIT SMOOTHIE BOWL

Serves: *3*

Prep Time: *5* Minutes

Cook Time: *5* Minutes

Total Time: *10* Minutes

INGREDIENTS

- 2 packets frozen dragon fruit
- ¼ cup frozen raspberries
- 2 bananas
- 2 tablespoons protein powder
- ½ cup dairy-free milk

DIRECTIONS

1. **In a blender add all ingredients and blend until smooth**
2. **Adjust flavor by adding more banana or dairy-free milk**
3. **Divide between serving bowl and top with granola and serve**

BANANA PANCAKES

Serves: **4**

Prep Time: **10** Minutes

Cook Time: **15** Minutes

Total Time: **25** Minutes

INGREDIENTS

- ¼ cup coconut flour
- 1 banana
- ¼ cup water
- 1 egg
- 1 tablespoon honey
- 1 tsp cinnamon
- ¼ tsp baking soda
- ½ tsp salt
- ¼ tablespoon vanilla extract
- 1 tablespoon coconut oil

DIRECTIONS

1. Place all ingredients in a bowl and mix using a hand mixer
2. In a skillet add coconut oil and pour ¼ cup batter

3. Cook for 1-2 minutes per side
4. When ready remove and serve with syrup

AQUAFABA GRANOLA

Serves: **12**

Prep Time: **10** Minutes

Cook Time: **25** Minutes

Total Time: **35** Minutes

INGREDIENTS

- 2 cups gluten-free rolled oats
- 1 cup chopped raw nuts
- ¼ cup shredded coconut
- 1 tablespoon chia seeds
- ½ cup coconut sugar
- ¼ tsp salt
- ¼ tsp cinnamon
- ½ cup aquafaba
- ½ cup maple syrup

- 1 tsp vanilla extract
- ½ cup blueberries

DIRECTIONS

1. Preheat oven to 325 F
2. In a bowl add oats, nuts, chia seeds, coconut, coconut sugar, cinnamon, salt and stir to combine
3. Add aquafaba to a mixing bowl and use a hand mixer
4. Add maple syrup and vanilla and pour aquafaba mixture over the dry ingredients
5. Spread the mixture onto a parchment paper and bake for 30-35 minutes
6. Add dried fruits and serve when ready

MORNING OATS

Serves: 2

Prep Time: 10 Minutes

Cook Time: 15 Minutes

Total Time: 25 Minutes

INGREDIENTS

- 1 cup oats
- 2 cup water
- 1 pinch salt
- 1 tablespoon flaxseed meal
- 1 tablespoon maple syrup
- ½ tsp ground cinnamon
- fruit compote

DIRECTIONS

1. In a saucepan add water, oats, cover and soak for 4-5 hours or overnight
2. Add a pinch of salt and bring to a boil
3. Reduce heat and cook for 10-12 minutes or until the water is almost absorbed
4. When they are ready remove from heat
5. Divide between serving bowl, top with chia seeds, banana, almond milk and serve

BANANA MUFFINS

Serves: **12**

Prep Time: **10** Minutes

Cook Time: **30** Minutes

Total Time: **40** Minutes

INGREDIENTS

- 1 cup almond flour
- 1 cup pecan pieces
- 1 tsp cinnamon
- ¼ tsp nutmeg
- ¼ tsp baking powder
- ½ tsp salt
- 2 bananas
- 1 tablespoon honey
- 2 eggs

DIRECTIONS

1. Preheat the oven to 400 F
2. In a food processor add pecan pieces, cinnamon, almond flour, nutmeg, baking powder, salt and process for 45-60 seconds

3. Mush bananas, add honey, eggs and mix well
4. Add the flour mixture to the egg mixture and mix well
5. Scoop the butter into 12 muffin cups
6. Bake for 22-25 minutes or until ready

CINNAMON PEANUT BUTTER

Serves: *12*

Prep Time: *10* Minutes

Cook Time: *10* Minutes

Total Time: *20* Minutes

INGREDIENTS

- 2 cups unsalted peanuts
- ½ tsp salt
- 2 tablespoons cinnamon
- ½ tsp powdered stevia
- 1 tablespoon avocado oil
- ½ cup raisins

DIRECTIONS

1. In a blender add peanuts and blend for 4-5 minutes
2. Add cinnamon, salt, sweetener and blend for another 30-60 seconds
3. Add raisins and blend for another 30 seconds
4. Add more cinnamon if necessary and serve

BANANA SPLITS

Serves: **4**

Prep Time: **5** Minutes

Cook Time: **5** Minutes

Total Time: **10** Minutes

INGREDIENTS

- 4 bananas
- ¼ cup nut butter
- ½ cup coconut yogurt
- ½ cup Rawnola

- ¼ cup berries
- 3 tsp hemp seeds
- ½ cup unsweetened coconut flakes

DIRECTIONS

1. Cut a slit down the center of each banana
2. Top with nut butter, rawnola, berries, coconut yogurt, hemp seeds and coconut flakes
3. When ready, serve fresh

5 MINUTE RAW-NOLA

Serves: *4*
Prep Time: *10* Minutes
Cook Time: *45* Minutes
Total Time: *55* Minutes

INGREDIENTS

- 1 cup raw walnuts

- 14-16 pitted dates
- 1 heaping tablespoon hemp seeds
- 1 heaping tablespoon flaxseed meal
- 1 tsp chia seeds
- ¼ cup unsweetened coconut
- ¼ cup gluten-free oats
- ¼ tsp cinnamon
- ¼ tsp maca powder
- 1 pinch salt
- 2 tablespoons cacao ribs
- ½ cup cacao powder
- 1 tsp vanilla extract

DIRECTIONS

1. In a blender add nuts, dates and blend for 5-6 minutes
2. Add remaining ingredients and mix well
3. Add cacao ribs, dried fruits, vanilla extract and cacao powder
4. Blend again, top with coconut yogurt and enjoy

ZUCCHINI BREAD

Serves: **12**

Prep Time: **10** Minutes

Cook Time: **60** Minutes

Total Time: **70** Minutes

INGREDIENTS

- 2 batches flax egg
- ½ cup applesauce
- ½ cup maple syrup
- ½ cup coconut sugar
- 1 tsp baking soda
- 1 tsp baking powder
- ½ tsp salt
- ¼ cup unsweetened cocoa powder
- ½ cup melted coconut oil
- ½ cup unsweetened almond milk
- 1 cup zucchini
- 1/3 cup gluten-free flour blend
- ½ cup almond flour
- ½ cup chocolate chips

DIRECTIONS

1. Preheat the oven to 350 F
2. In a bowl mix flax eggs add maple syrup, coconut sugar, applesauce, baking soda, baking powder, cocoa powder, salt and whisk well
3. Add coconut oil, almond milk, grated zucchini and stir to combine
4. Add out flour, almond flour, and stir in chocolate chips
5. Transfer batter to the loaf pan and top with a couple of chocolate chips
6. Bake for 45-55 minutes or until done
7. When ready remove and serve

PEANUT BUTTER & ACAI BOWLS

Serves: 4
Prep Time: 10   Minutes
Cook Time: 15   Minutes
Total Time: 25   Minutes

INGREDIENTS

- 2 packets unsweetened acai
- 1 banana
- 2 tablespoons peanut butter powder
- ½ cup unsweetened coconut
- 1 cup spinach
- ½ cup mixed berries

TOPPINGS

- ½ banana
- 1 tablespoon unsweetened coconut
- 2 tablespoons sunflower seeds

DIRECTIONS

1. In a blender add acai, dairy-free milk, peanut butter powder, spinach and blend until smooth
2. Blend until the mixture is thick
3. Adjust flavor by adding peanut butter powder
4. Divide between 2 serving bowls garnish with toppings and serve

DARK CHOCOLATE GRANOLA

Serves: **8**

Prep Time: **10** Minutes

Cook Time: **25** Minutes

Total Time: **35** Minutes

INGREDIENTS

- 2 cups gluten free rolled oats
- 1 cup chopped raw nuts
- ½ cup shredded coconut
- 2 tablespoons chia seeds
- 2 tablespoons coconut sugar
- 1 tsp salt
- ½ cup cocoa powder
- ½ cup coconut oil
- ¼ cup maple syrup
- ¼ cup dark chocolate chips

DIRECTIONS

1. Preheat the oven to 350 F

2. In a blender add coconut, chia seeds, nuts, oats, salt, coconut sugar and cocoa powder and blend until smooth
3. In a saucepan add coconut oil, maple syrup and pour melted mixture over the dry ingredients and mix well
4. Spread the mixture onto a baking sheet and bake for 20-25 minutes or until golden brown
5. When ready remove from the oven and serve

POTATO HASH BROWNS

Serves: 4

Prep Time: 10 Minutes

Cook Time: 20 Minutes

Total Time: 30 Minutes

INGREDIENTS

- 2 sweet potatoes
- 1 tablespoon avocado oil
- 1 pinch of salt
- 1 pinch of pepper

DIRECTIONS

1. Spiralize your potatoes into thin noodles
2. In a skillet add olive oil, sweet potatoes and season with salt and pepper
3. Cook for 8-10 minutes or until crispy
4. When ready, serve with herbs or hot sauce

BANANA NUT BUTTER PANCAKES

Serves: *4*
Prep Time: *10* Minutes
Cook Time: *20* Minutes
Total Time: *30* Minutes

INGREDIENTS

- 2 bananas
- ¼ cup pecan butter
- 3 eggs
- 1 tsp baking soda

DIRECTIONS

1. In a bowl mix all pancake ingredients
2. Pour batter in a greased skillet
3. Cook for 1-2 minutes per side and serve with strawberry syrup

BREAKFAST MUFFINS

Serves: 2

Prep Time: 10 Minutes

Cook Time: 30 Minutes

Total Time: 40 Minutes

INGREDIENTS

- 2 eggs
- ½ cup yogurt
- 2 tablespoons olive oil
- ¼ lb. apple sauce
- 1 banana

- 3 tablespoons honey
- 1 tsp vanilla extract
- ½ lb. whole meal flour
- 2 oz. oats
- 1 tsp baking powder
- 1 tsp cinnamon
- ¼ lb. blueberry

DIRECTIONS

1. Preheat oven to 300 F
2. In a bowl mix all ingredients
3. Pour batter into 12 large muffin cases
4. Sprinkle with extra oats and seeds
5. Bake for 22-25 minutes or until golden brown
6. When ready remove and serve

ZUCCHINI BANANA MUFFINS

Serves: **4**

Prep Time: **10** Minutes

Cook Time: **15** Minutes

Total Time: **25** Minutes

INGREDIENTS

- 2 bananas
- 1 zucchini
- 1 egg
- ½ cup nut butter
- 1 tsp cinnamon
- ¾ shredded unsweetened coconut
- ¼ cup almond flour
- ¼ tsp salt

DIRECTIONS

1. **Preheat the oven to 350 F**
2. **In a bowl mash the bananas**
3. **Add grated zucchini, egg, nut butter and mix well**
4. **Stir in coconut, almond flour, salt, cinnamon, and mix well**

5. Fill each muffin tin with a ¼ cup of the mixture
6. Bake for 12-15 minutes
7. When ready, remove and serve

GLUTEN-FREE PANCAKES

Serves: **6**

Prep Time: **10** Minutes

Cook Time: **10** Minutes

Total Time: **20** Minutes

INGREDIENTS

- 1 cup gluten-free flour blend
- 1 cup buttermilk
- 1 egg
- 1 tablespoon sugar
- 2 tablespoons unsalted butter
- 2 tsp gluten-free baking powder
- ½ tsp salt
- maple syrup

DIRECTIONS

1. In a bowl mix all ingredients until smooth
2. Heat a griddle to 325 F
3. Spoon ¼ cup batter onto griddle and cook for 1-2 minutes per side
4. When ready remove and serve with syrup

CINNAMON WAFFLES

Serves: 5

Prep Time: 10 Minutes

Cook Time: 20 Minutes

Total Time: 30 Minutes

INGREDIENTS

- 1 cup low-fat yogurt
- ½ cup nonfat milk
- 1 egg
- 1 tablespoon honey

- 1 tablespoon butter
- 1 cup whole wheat flour
- 2 tsp baking powder
- 1 tsp cinnamon

DIRECTIONS

1. Preheat waffle iron
2. In a bowl mix all ingredients for the waffles
3. Pour ¼ cup batter into waffle iron and cook according to the instructions
4. When ready remove and serve with maple syrup or honey

CHEESE GRIT MUFFINS

Serves: **12**
Prep Time: **15** Minutes
Cook Time: **45** Minutes
Total Time: **60** Minutes

INGREDIENTS

- 1 cup all-purpose flour
- 1 tsp baking powder
- ¼ tsp baking soda
- ¼ tsp salt
- 1 egg
- 1/3 cup buttermilk
- ½ cup butter
- 1 cup grits
- 1 cup grated cheddar cheese
- 1 tablespoon fresh chives

DIRECTIONS

1. Preheat oven to 325 F and grease a 12 cups of muffin pan with butter
2. In a bowl mix all ingredients for muffins
3. Stir in cheese, chives and spoon batter into muffin cups
4. Bake for 30 minutes or until muffins are golden brown
5. When ready, remove and serve

CHOCHOLATE OATMEAL

Serves: **3**

Prep Time: **10** Minutes

Cook Time: **25** Minutes

Total Time: **35** Minutes

INGREDIENTS

- 1 cup low-fat yogurt
- ½ cup low-fat chocolate milk
- 1 tablespoon creamy peanut butter
- 1 cup oat-fashioned oats
- ¼ cup strawberries

DIRECTIONS

1. In a bowl combine chocolate milk, peanut butter, oats, yogurt and stir well
2. Divide mixture among 4 serving size containers
3. Top with strawberries and serve

DESSERTS

SPRINGTIME AVOCADO

Serves: 2
Prep Time: 5 Minutes
Cook Time: 5 Minutes
Total Time: 10 Minutes

INGREDIENTS

- ½ cup low-fat yogurt
- 2 tablespoons chives
- 2 tablespoons olive oil
- ½ tsp salt
- 1 Matzah sheet
- 1 avocado
- 2 radishes

DIRECTIONS

1. In a bowl combine oil, yogurt, chives, salt and spread mixture on the Matzah
2. Arrange radishes and avocado on top of the Matzzah
3. Drizzle with oil, thyme, salt and serve

APPLE YOGURT PARFAIT

Serves: **4**

Prep Time: **10** Minutes

Cook Time: **10** Minutes

Total Time: **20** Minutes

INGREDIENTS

- 1 apple
- 1 cup bran flakes
- 1 cup low-fat yogurt

DIRECTIONS

1. In a glass add yogurt, cup brand flakes and apples
2. Top with yogurt and sprinkle with cinnamon
3. Serve when ready

YOGURT POPS

Serves: **6**

Prep Time: **5** Minutes

Cook Time: **5** Minutes

Total Time: **10** Minutes

INGREDIENTS

- 1 cup low-fat yogurt
- 1 cup strawberries
- ¼ cup chopped kiwi
- ¼ cup blueberries
- 6 paper cuts
- 6 wooden popsicle sticks

DIRECTIONS

1. **In a bowl place yogurt and stir in fruits**
2. **Divide mixture into 6-8 paper cups**
3. **Place popsicle stick in each cup**
4. **Freeze overnight and serve next morning**

CHOCOLATE CHEESECAKES

Serves: **6**

Prep Time: **10** Minutes

Cook Time: **120** Minutes

Total Time: **130** Minutes

INGREDIENTS

- 6 chocolate wafer cookies
- 3 oz. cream cheese
- ¼ cup low-fat yogurt
- ½ cup sugar
- 1 egg
- 1 tablespoon cocoa powder
- 1 tsp vanilla extract
- ¼ cup chocolate chips

DIRECTIONS

1. Preheat oven to 325 F
2. Place 6-8 cupcake liners into muffin tin
3. Place a wafer cookie into each cupcake liner
4. In a blender add cream cheese, sugar, egg yogurt, vanilla and blend until smooth

5. Add melted chocolate and divide butter among the muffin cups
6. Bake for 18-20 minutes, when ready remove and garnish with raspberries

LUSCIOUS LEMON PARFAIT

Serves: **6**

Prep Time: **10** Minutes

Cook Time: **30** Minutes

Total Time: **40** Minutes

INGREDIENTS

- 1 qt. low-fat vanilla yogurt
- 1/3 cup lemon curd
- 1 cup graham crackers
- ¾ cup toasted coconut

DIRECTIONS

1. Into each parfait glass add yogurt, lemon curd, coconut and graham crackers
2. Serve when ready

PUMPKIN CARAMEL CAKE

Serves: 8

Prep Time: 10 Minutes

Cook Time: 45 Minutes

Total Time: 55 Minutes

INGREDIENTS

- ¼ cup honey
- 1 cup pumpkin puree
- 2 sticks butter
- 4 eggs
- ¼ cup coconut flour
- 1 cup almond flour
- ¼ tsp salt
- 1 tablespoon cinnamon

- ¼ tsp ginger
- ½ tsp nutmeg
- 1 tsp baking soda

DIRECTIONS

1. In a bowl mix all ingredients until fully incorporated
2. Pour into a greased cake pan
3. Bake at 375 F for 40-45 minutes
4. When ready, remove pour caramel sauce and serve

BLACK BEAN BROWNIES

Serves: *12*

Prep Time: *5* Minutes

Cook Time: *15* Minutes

Total Time: *20* Minutes

INGREDIENTS

- 1 can black beans

- 1 tablespoon cocoa powder
- ¼ cup oats
- ½ tsp salt
- ¼ cup maple syrup
- ½ cup coconut oil
- 1 tsp vanilla extract
- ¼ tsp baking powder
- ¼ cup chocolate chips

DIRECTIONS

1. Preheat oven to 325 F
2. In a blender add all ingredients and blend until smooth
3. Stir in chocolate chips and pour mixture into a pan
4. Bake for 20-25 minutes or until olden brown
5. When ready remove from the oven and serve

BLUEBERRY BITES

Serves: **8**

Prep Time: **10** Minutes

Cook Time: **50** Minutes

Total Time: **60** Minutes

INGREDIENTS

- 2 cup old-fashioned oats
- ¼ cup almond butter
- ½ cup honey
- 1 tsp vanilla
- ¼ tsp cinnamon
- 1 cup blueberries

DIRECTIONS

1. In a bowl combine almond butter, honey, oats, cinnamon and vanilla
2. Fold in blueberries and mix well
3. Refrigerate for 45-60 minutes
4. Mold mixture into balls and serve

APPLE PIE COOKIES

Serves: **12**

Prep Time: **10** Minutes

Cook Time: **50** Minutes

Total Time: **60** Minutes

INGREDIENTS

- 1 cup oats
- 1/3 cup whole wheat flour
- 1 tsp baking powder
- 1 tsp cinnamon
- ¼ tsp salt
- 1 tablespoon coconut oil
- 1 egg
- 1 tsp vanilla extract
- ¼ cup honey
- 1 cup red apple

DIRECTIONS

1. In a bowl mix all dry and wet ingredients together
2. Refrigerate dough for 20-30 minutes
3. Preheat the oven to 350 F

4. Divide dough into 12-14 cookies on onto a baking sheet
5. Bake for 12-15 minutes
6. When ready remove and serve

RICE BARS

Serves: **12**

Prep Time: **10** Minutes

Cook Time: **60** Minutes

Total Time: **70** Minutes

INGREDIENTS

- 4 cups gluten-free rice cereal
- ¼ cup peanut butter
- 1/3 cup honey
- dash of salt
- 1 tsp vanilla extract
- 2 tablespoons melted chocolate

DIRECTIONS

1. In a bowl combine all ingredients except chocolate
2. Spread the mixture across a prepared pan and press it down into the pan
3. Drizzle melted chocolate over the bars
4. Refrigerate for 50-60 minutes
5. When ready remove and serve

SMOOTHIES

BANANA SMOOTHIE

Serves: **1**

Prep Time: **5** Minutes

Cook Time: **5** Minutes

Total Time: **10** Minutes

INGREDIENTS

- ¼ cup strawberries
- ½ banana
- 1 orange
- 1 cup ice

DIRECTIONS

1. **In a blender place all ingredients and blend until smooth**
2. **Pour smoothie in a glass and serve**

LIVER DETOX SMOOTHIE

Serves: **1**

Prep Time: **5** Minutes

Cook Time: **5** Minutes

Total Time: **10** Minutes

INGREDIENTS

- 1 banana
- ¼ green apple
- 1 carrot
- 1 handful baby spinach
- 1 tablespoon parsley
- 2 walnut halves
- 2 tablespoons protein powder
- ¼ lemon juice
- 1 pinch cinnamon

DIRECTIONS

1. **In a blender place all ingredients and blend until smooth**
2. **Pour smoothie in a glass and serve**

GREEN PROTEIN SMOOTHIE

Serves: *1*

Prep Time: *5* Minutes

Cook Time: *5* Minutes

Total Time: *10* Minutes

INGREDIENTS

- 1 banana
- 1 handful baby spinach
- 1 cup unsweetened almond milk
- 1 tablespoon unsweetened almond butter
- ½ cup plain yogurt
- ¼ tsp Maca powder
- 1 tsp cinnamon

DIRECTIONS

1. **In a blender place all ingredients and blend until smooth**
2. **Pour smoothie in a glass and serve**

CITRUS LIVER BOOST SMOOTHIE

Serves: *1*
Prep Time: *5* Minutes
Cook Time: *5* Minutes
Total Time: *10* Minutes

INGREDIENTS

- 2 oranges
- 1 lemon
- ¼ cup greens
- 1 rib celery
- ¼ cup parsley
- 1 cup water

DIRECTIONS

1. In a blender place all ingredients and blend until smooth
2. Pour smoothie in a glass and serve

LIVER GREEN SMOOTHIE

Serves: *1*

Prep Time: *5* Minutes

Cook Time: *5* Minutes

Total Time: *10* Minutes

INGREDIENTS

- ½ cup spinach
- ¼ cup arugula
- 2 stalks celery
- juice from 1 lemon
- water if necessary

DIRECTIONS

1. **In a blender place all ingredients and blend until smooth**
2. **Pour smoothie in a glass and serve**

ARTICHOKE SMOOTHIE

Serves: **1**

Prep Time: **5** Minutes

Cook Time: **5** Minutes

Total Time: **10** Minutes

INGREDIENTS

- 1 cup artichoke hearts
- 1 cup spinach
- 1 clove garlic
- 1 pinch of turmeric
- juice of ¼ lemon

DIRECTIONS

1. In a blender place all ingredients and blend until smooth
2. Pour smoothie in a glass and serve

KALE LIVER DETOX SMOOTHIE

Serves: 1

Prep Time: 5 Minutes

Cook Time: 5 Minutes

Total Time: 10 Minutes

INGREDIENTS

- 1 cup Kale
- 1 apple
- 1 lemon
- 1-inch ginger
- 1 cup water

DIRECTIONS

1. In a blender place all ingredients and blend until smooth
2. Pour smoothie in a glass and serve

ZUCCHINI LIVER DETOX SMOOTHIE

Serves: **1**
Prep Time: **5** Minutes
Cook Time: **5** Minutes
Total Time: **10** Minutes

INGREDIENTS

- 1 apple
- 1 zucchini
- ½ avocado
- 1 cup greens
- ½ cup coriander
- ½ tsp turmeric
- juice of ½ lemon
- 1 cup coconut water

DIRECTIONS

1. **In a blender place all ingredients and blend until smooth**
2. **Pour smoothie in a glass and serve**

SPRING LIVER DETOX SMOOTHIE

Serves: *1*

Prep Time: *5* Minutes

Cook Time: *5* Minutes

Total Time: *10* Minutes

INGREDIENTS

- 2 beets
- 2 carrots
- 1 cup dandelion greens
- 1 lemon
- 1 apple
- 1 cup cabbage
- 2 tablespoons protein powder

DIRECTIONS

1. In a blender place all ingredients and blend until smooth
2. Pour smoothie in a glass and serve

STRAWBERRY MORNING SMOOTHIE

Serves: *1*

Prep Time: *5* Minutes

Cook Time: *5* Minutes

Total Time: *10* Minutes

INGREDIENTS

- ½ cup coconut milk
- 1/4 banana
- 5-6 strawberries
- ½ cup gluten-free oats
- ¼ tsp vanilla extract

DIRECTIONS

1. In a blender place all ingredients and blend until smooth
2. Pour smoothie in a glass and serve

LIVER ENERGY BOOSTING SMOOTHIE

Serves: **1**

Prep Time: **5** Minutes

Cook Time: **5** Minutes

Total Time: **10** Minutes

INGREDIENTS

- 3 stalks celery
- ½ cup parsley
- 1 tsp Spirulina
- juice of ½ lemon

DIRECTIONS

1. **In a blender place all ingredients and blend until smooth**
2. **Pour smoothie in a glass and serve**

PAPAYA LIVER SMOOTHIE

Serves: *1*
Prep Time: *5* Minutes
Cook Time: *5* Minutes
Total Time: *10* Minutes

INGREDIENTS

- 2 cups papaya
- 1 tablespoon papaya seeds
- juice of ½ lime
- 1 cup water

DIRECTIONS

1. In a blender place all ingredients and blend until smooth
2. Pour smoothie in a glass and serve

LIVER BLUEBERRIES SMOOTHIE

Serves: 1
Prep Time: 5 Minutes
Cook Time: 5 Minutes
Total Time: 10 Minutes

INGREDIENTS

- ½ cup blueberries
- ¼ cup red cabbage
- ¼ grapefruit
- 1 tablespoon ginger
- 1 cup coconut water

DIRECTIONS

1. **In a blender place all ingredients and blend until smooth**
2. **Pour smoothie in a glass and serve**

TURMERIC LIVER SMOOTHIE

Serves: *1*

Prep Time: *5* Minutes

Cook Time: *5* Minutes

Total Time: *10* Minutes

INGREDIENTS

- 1 tablespoon turmeric grated
- 1 cup kale
- 1 apple
- 1 cup berries
- 1 cup almond milk

DIRECTIONS

1. **In a blender place all ingredients and blend until smooth**
2. **Pour smoothie in a glass and serve**

BEETROOT LIVER DETOX SMOOTHIE

Serves: *1*

Prep Time: *5* Minutes

Cook Time: *5* Minutes

Total Time: *10* Minutes

INGREDIENTS

- 1 cup coconut water
- 1 cup strawberries
- 1 beetroot
- 1 tablespoon chia seeds

DIRECTIONS

1. In a blender place all ingredients and blend until smooth
2. Pour smoothie in a glass and serve

CARROT & BEETROOT SMOOTHIE

Serves: *1*

Prep Time: *5* Minutes

Cook Time: *5* Minutes

Total Time: *10* Minutes

INGREDIENTS

- 1 beetroot grated
- 1 cup carrot juice
- 1 apple
- 1 tablespoon ginger
- 1/3 cup cilantro
- ¼ cup coconut water

DIRECTIONS

1. **In a blender place all ingredients and blend until smooth**
2. **Pour smoothie in a glass and serve**

SPINACH LIVER DETOX SMOOTHIE

Serves: *1*

Prep Time: *5* Minutes

Cook Time: *5* Minutes

Total Time: *10* Minutes

INGREDIENTS

- 1 cucumber
- 1 cup spinach
- 1 lemon
- 1 cup Swiss chard
- 1 cup water

DIRECTIONS

1. **In a blender place all ingredients and blend until smooth**
2. **Pour smoothie in a glass and serve**

APPLE CIDER SMOOTHIE

Serves: **1**

Prep Time: **5** Minutes

Cook Time: **5** Minutes

Total Time: **10** Minutes

INGREDIENTS

- 1 tablespoon apple cider vinegar
- 1 tablespoon lemon juice
- 1 tsp turmeric
- 1 cup water
- ½ tablespoon maple syrup
- ¼ cup pineapple

DIRECTIONS

1. In a blender place all ingredients and blend until smooth
2. Pour smoothie in a glass and serve

GRAPEFRUIT SMOOTHIE

Serves: *1*

Prep Time: *5* Minutes

Cook Time: *5* Minutes

Total Time: *10* Minutes

INGREDIENTS

- 1 grapefruit
- 1 lemon
- 1 cup water
- ½ cucumber
- 1 avocado
- 1 clove garlic
- 1-inch ginger

DIRECTIONS

1. **In a blender place all ingredients and blend until smooth**
2. **Pour smoothie in a glass and serve**

KIWI SMOOTHIE

Serves: **1**

Prep Time: **5** Minutes

Cook Time: **5** Minutes

Total Time: **10** Minutes

INGREDIENTS

- 1 cup almond milk
- 2 kiwi fruits
- 1 banana
- ¼ cup silken tofu
- ¼ cup oats
- ¼ tsp ginger
-

DIRECTIONS

1. In a blender place all ingredients and blend until smooth
2. Pour smoothie in a glass and serve

Made in United States
Orlando, FL
03 November 2023